EMERGING CONCEPTS OF PHYSIOTHERAPY

NIHAR RANJAN MOHANTY

Copyright © NIHAR RANJAN MOHANTY
All Rights Reserved.

ISBN 978-1-64733-096-5

This book has been published with all efforts taken to make the material error-free after the consent of the author. However, the author and the publisher do not assume and hereby disclaim any liability to any party for any loss, damage, or disruption caused by errors or omissions, whether such errors or omissions result from negligence, accident, or any other cause.

While every effort has been made to avoid any mistake or omission, this publication is being sold on the condition and understanding that neither the author nor the publishers or printers would be liable in any manner to any person by reason of any mistake or omission in this publication or for any action taken or omitted to be taken or advice rendered or accepted on the basis of this work. For any defect in printing or binding the publishers will be liable only to replace the defective copy by another copy of this work then available.

DEDICATED TO MY BELOVED PARENTS

Contents

Preface — *vii*

Acknowledgements — *ix*

1. Introduction — 1
2. Physiotherapeutic Interventions — 13
3. Therapeutic Approaches In Various Conditions — 31
4. Physiotherapy In Women's Health — 55
5. Bibliography — 110

Preface

This book is a simplified form to describe various approaches and therapeutic interventions of physiotherapy. This book is divided into five chapters. Students and researchers of physical therapy can get the information related to basic and emerging aspects of physiotherapy ready hand from this book. The language is lucid and written in a very concise manner. Point-wise presentation of the subject matters is the strength of this book. Concise and informative matters of the subject are the motto of this book.

Acknowledgements

First and foremost I would like to thank the almighty for his support and blessings in this long journey.

I would like to express my deepest sense of gratitude to my respected teacher & guide, **Prof. (Dr.) Shyamal Koley**, Head, Department of Physiotherapy, Guru Nanak Dev University, Amritsar, whose knowledge, guidance, and constant encouragement and deep insight without which this book would not have found its final shape.

I would like to thank my **Mother**, for all her support, guidance, motivation and unconditional love, without which I would have never made it through my book. Along with her my greatest regards goes to my **Father, my sisters and my brothers** for the confidence they had in me and I am at loss of words to convey my appreciation and warm regards to them.

My sincere thanks go to my friends **Avinash Tiwari** for helping me in my book and being with me in need.

Nihar Ranjan Mohanty

EMERGING CONCEPTS OF PHYSIOTHERAPY

Nihar Ranjan Mohanty
BPT; [SWAMI VIVEKANAND NATIONAL INSTITUTE OF REHABILITATION TRAINING AND RESEARCH, Cuttack, Odisha, India]
MPT (Sports); [GURU NANAK DEV UNIVERSITY, Amritsar, Punjab, India]

CHAPTER ONE

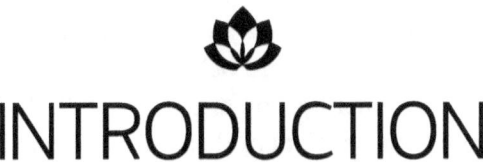

INTRODUCTION

Physiotherapists have different titles in different countries: in many countries they are called physical therapists. Some countries have their own version of the word physiotherapist, such as kinesiologist. They are all part of the same profession.

According to **WCPT** "**Physical therapists** provide services that develop, maintain and restore people's maximum movement and functional ability. They can help people at any stage of life, when movement and function are threatened by ageing, injury, diseases, disorders, conditions or environmental factors. Physical therapists help people maximise their quality of life, looking at physical, psychological, emotional and social wellbeing. They work in the health spheres of promotion, prevention, treatment/intervention, rehabilitation."

According to **WHO** "**Physiotherapists** assess, plan and implement rehabilitative programs that improve or restore human motor functions, maximize movement ability, relieve pain syndromes, and treat or prevent physical challenges associated with injuries, diseases and other impairments. They apply a broad range of physical therapies and techniques such as movement, ultrasound, heating, laser and other techniques. They may develop and implement programmes for screening and prevention of common physical ailments and disorders."

Role of Physiotherapist in community

- Assess physical condition of patients to identify problems and plan appropriate treatment
- Perform spinal and peripheral joint mobilisation and manipulation (where appropriate)
- Assist in the reduction of pain and swelling, improve the range of movement, assist in muscle re-education and strengthening through the

use of equipment/techniques such as hot/cold packs, electrotherapy, manual therapy, biofeedback, taping and splinting
- Retrain patients to walk or use devices such as walking frames, crutches, sticks, wheelchairs, splints to assist/improve mobility
- Assess development of premature babies and plan and provide therapy for children with movement problems/physical disabilities
- Assist individuals with permanent disabilities to maximise their ability to function as optimally as possible and to manage the physical demands of daily living
- Work as part of a team of health professionals, to provide a multidisciplinary care plan, to improve a person's health
- Educate patients, their families, industry and the community to lead healthy lifestyles and to prevent injury and disability
- Plan and implement community fitness/exercise programs, including hydrotherapy programs for people both with and without a disability
- Maintain relevant documentation associated with patient care eg. Patient records, reports, statistics.
- Conduct re-examinations
- Modify interventions as necessary to achieve anticipated goals and expected outcomes

COMMON TERMINOLOGIES

Impairment — is a problem "in body function or structure as a significant deviation or loss"; is the manifestation of an underlying pathology; can be temporary or permanent, progressive, regressive or static, intermittent or continuous, slight through too severe

Disability — is the umbrella term for impairments, activity limitations, and participation restrictions that results from the interaction between an individual's health condition and the personal and environmental contextual factors. Personal factors are the particular background of an individual's life and living, and comprise features of the individual that are not part of a health condition or health states, such as: gender, race age, fitness, lifestyle, habits, coping styles, social background, education, profession, past and current experience, overall behaviour pattern, character style, individual psychological assets, and other characteristics, all or any of which may play a role in disability in any level. Environmental factors are external factors that make up the physical, social and attitudinal environment in which people live and conduct their lives. Disability can be described at three levels: body (impairment of body function or structure), person (activity limitations), and society (participation restrictions).

A disability is any continuing condition that restricts everyday activities. Disabilities can affect a person's capacity to communicate, interact with others, learn and get about independently. Disability is usually permanent but may be episodic (WA Disability Services Act 1993).

Types of disability
Disabilities can be:
Sensory: affecting vision and / or hearing.
Neurological: affecting a person's ability to control their movements.
Physical: affecting mobility and/or a person's ability to use their upper or lower body. These generally relate to the musculoskeletal, circulatory, respiratory and nervous systems.
Intellectual: these can include intellectual and developmental disabilities which can relate to difficulties with thought processes, learning, communicating, remembering information and using it appropriately, making judgements and problem solving.
Cognitive: affecting a person's thought processes, personality and memory resulting, for example, from an injury to the brain.
Psychiatric: affecting a person's emotions, thought processes and behaviour.

Some disabilities, such as epilepsy, are hidden, while others, such as cerebral palsy, may be visible.

People may have more than one disability and may experience additional disadvantages to adequate service provision due to factors such as being from culturally and linguistically diverse backgrounds or because they live outside the metropolitan area or outside a regional centre.

Causes of disability

The causes of disability vary. As a person ages the severity of the disability can change.
Disabilities may be:

- Genetically determined;
- Environmentally determined; or
- Unknown cause.

A genetically determined disability is usually inherited from the parents. However, a new genetic error can occur leading to symptoms of the condition. Examples of this are cystic fibrosis and muscular dystrophy.

An environmentally determined disability results from an accident, injury, disease or infection. Examples include acquired brain injury, spinal cord injury and diabetes.

Sometimes a disability is of unknown origin. This is the case with many physical and intellectual disabilities.

Disabilities vary according to individual circumstances.

The impact of disability

While the degree and type of disability varies with individual circumstances, people with disabilities frequently report that they experience difficulty being independently mobile, or being able to see, hear, or communicate.

As a consequence, people with disabilities face barriers with everyday activities such as hearing or understanding what is said, seeing small print, climbing stairs or understanding signage.

The impact on the life of the person concerned can be major, particularly if the individual has multiple disabilities. Often people with disabilities are unable to do things most of us take for granted, such as:

- reading and understanding public notices or newsletters;
- accessing websites;
- participating at the local swimming pool or recreation centre;
- playing on the play equipment at the park;
- hearing what is said at a public meeting; and
- Shopping at the local shops.

The exact impact of a disability on the life of an individual varies according to a number of factors including:

- the specific nature and severity of the disability;
- the person's strength, stamina, size, weight and age;
- the person's ability to cope; and
- The physical, social and economic environment within which the person is living.

Communities which are accessible and inclusive minimises the effect of disability.

Disability

Disability is part of the human condition. Almost everyone will be temporarily or permanently impaired at some point in life, and those who survive to old age will experience increasing difficulties in functioning. Most extended families have a disabled member, and many non-disabled people take responsibility for supporting and caring for their relatives and friends with disabilities.

"disability results from the interaction between persons with impairments and attitudinal and environmental barriers that hinder their full and effective participation in society on an equal basis with others".

As a result of impairment may involve difficulties in walking, seeing, speaking, hearing, reading, writing, counting, lifting, or taking interest in and making one's surrounding.

- **Temporary Total Disability** - Period in which the affected person is totally unable to work. During this period, he may receive orthopaedic, opthalmological, auditory or speech any other medical treatment.
- Temporary **partialDisability** - Period when recovery has reached the stage of improvement so that person may began some kind of gainful occupation.
- **Permanent Disability** - Permanent damage or loss of use of some part/parts of the body after the stage of maximum improvement [from any medical treatment] has been reached and the condition is stationary.

Environment

A person's environment has a huge impact on the experience and extent of disability. Inaccessible environments create disability by creating barriers to participation and inclusion. Examples of the possible negative impact of the environment include:

- a Deaf individual without a sign language interpreter
- a wheelchair user in a building without an accessible bathroom or elevator
- a blind person using a computer without screen-reading software.

Health is also affected by environmental factors, such as safe water and sanitation, nutrition, poverty, working conditions, climate, or access to health care.

The environment may be changed to improve health conditions, prevent impairments, and improve outcomes for persons with disabilities. Such changes can be brought about by legislation, policy changes, capacity building, or technological developments leading to, for instance:

- accessible design of the built environment and transport;
- signage to benefit people with sensory impairments;
- more accessible health, rehabilitation, education, and support services;
- more opportunities for work and employment for persons with disabilities.

The International Classification of Functioning, problems with human functioning is categorized in three interconnected areas:

- impairments are problems in body function or alterations in body structure – for example, paralysis or blindness;
- activity limitations are difficulties in executing activities – for example, walking or eating;
- participation restrictions are problems with involvement in any area of life – for example, facing discrimination in employment or transportation.

Disability refers to difficulties encountered in any or all three areas of functioning. The ICF can also be used to understand and measure the positive aspects of functioning such as body functions, activities, participation and environmental facilitation. The ICF adopts neutral language and does not distinguish between the type and cause of disability – for instance, between "physical" and "mental" health. "Health conditions" are diseases, injuries, and disorders, while "impairments" are specific decrements in body functions and structures, often identified as symptoms or signs of health conditions.

Disability arises from the interaction of health conditions with contextual factors – environmental and personal factors as shown in the figure below.

The ICF contains a classification of **environmental factors** describing the world in which people with different levels of functioning must live and act. These factors can be either facilitators or barriers. Environmental factors include: products and technology; the natural and built environment; support and relationships; attitudes; and services, systems, and policies.

The ICF also recognizes **personal factors**, such as motivation and self-esteem, which can influence how much a person participates in society. However, these factors are not yet conceptualized or classified. It further distinguishes between a person's **capacities** to perform actions and the actual **performance** of those actions in real life, a subtle difference that helps illuminate the effect of environment and how performance might be improved by modifying the environment.

Prevention

Prevention of health conditions associated with disability is a development issue. Attention to environmental factors – including nutrition, preventable diseases, safe water and sanitation, safety on roads and in workplaces – can greatly reduce the incidence of health conditions leading to disability.

A public health approach distinguishes:

Primary prevention – actions to avoid or remove the cause of a health problem in an individual or a population before it arises. It includes health promotion and specific protection (for example, HIV education).

Secondary prevention – actions to detect a health problem at an early stage in an individual or a population, facilitating cure, or reducing or preventing spread, or reducing or preventing its long-term effects (for example, supporting women with intellectual disability to access breast cancer screening).

Tertiary prevention – actions to reduce the impact of an already established disease by restoring function and reducing disease-related complications (for example, rehabilitation for children with musculoskeletal impairment).

Rehabilitation definedas "a set of measures that assist individuals who experience, or are likely to experience, disability to achieve and maintain optimal functioning in interaction with their environments". A distinction is sometimes made between habilitation, which aims to help those who acquire disabilities congenitally or early in life to develop maximal functioning; and rehabilitation, where those who have experienced a loss in function are assisted to regain maximal functioning. Rehabilitation involves identification of a person's problems and needs, relating the problems to relevant factors of the person and the environment, defining rehabilitation goals, planning and implementing the measures, and assessing the effects (see figure below).

Prevention of Disabilities

1. *Prevention at three levels*
2. *General Preventive Measures*
3. *Care During Pregnancy*
4. *Care at the time of birth*
5. *Early Childhood Care*

1. **Prevention at three levels**

- Primary Prevention
- Secondary Prevention
- Tertiary Prevention

2. **General Preventive Measures**

i. Marriage between very close blood relations like uncle, niece, first cousin should be avoided for prevention of hereditary disorders.
ii. Avoid pregnancies before the age of 18 years and after the age of 35 years.
iii. Consult a doctor before planning the pregnancy;

- If there is incidence of birth defects in your family.
- If you have had difficulty in conceiving or have had a series of miscarriages, still births, twins, delivery by operation (Caesarean), obstructed labour/prolonged labour(more than 12 hours) and/or severe bleeding in previous pregnancy .
- If you have RH - negative blood type.
- If you have diabetes.

3. **Care during Pregnancy**

I. Avoid hard physical work such as carrying heavy loads, especially in fields, and other accident - prone activities such as walking on slippery ground or climbing stools and chairs.
II. Avoid unnecessary drugs and medications. Even the normally considered safe drugs which are sold commonly can potentially cause serious defects in an unborn child.
III. Avoid smoking, chewing tobacco, consuming alcohol and narcotics.
IV. Avoid X - rays, and exposure to any kind of radiation.
V. Avoid exposure to illnesses like measles, mumps etc, especially during the first 3 months of pregnancy.
VI. Avoid sexual contact with a person having venereal disease.
VII. Take precautions against lead poisoning.
VIII. Avoid too much use of 'Surma' and 'Kohl'.
IX. Eat a well-balanced and nourishing diet supplemented with green leafy vegetables, proteins and vitamins.
X. All women of the child bearing age need 0.4mg of folic acid daily. It is also available in folic acid plus iron tablets which should be taken for at least 3 months during the third trimester when the risk of developing iron deficiency anemia is greatest.
XI. Ensure weight gain of at last 10 kgs. Have regular medical checkups.
XII. All pregnant women should be given tetanus injection.
XIII. Woman at 'high - risk', whose weight is < 38 Kg, height is less than 152 cm, weight gain during pregnancy <6 kg or who is severly anaemia c (Hb < 8mg), having frequent pregnancies, having a history of miscarriage/abortion/premature deliveries, must get expert prenatal care so as to have a normal baby.
XIV. Must consult a doctor, in case of edema (swelling) of feet, persistent headache, fever, difficulty or pain in passing urine, bleeding from the vagina, and yellowness of eyes (jaundice)

4. **Care at the time of birth**

I. Delivery must be conducted by trained personnel, preferably in a hospital where all facilities are available.
II. If a baby does not cry immediately after birth, resuscitation measures should be undertaken at once.
III. Babies born prematurely and with a low birth weight (<2.5 Kg) may need Neonatal Intensive Care.

IV. If the baby's head appears to be abnormally small or large then a physician should be consulted, preferably a pediatrician. The approximate head size for a male child at birth is 35 cm and for female child is 34.5 cm.
V. To protect a child from infections, breast - feeding must be started immediately after birth. First milk (colostrum) must be fed to the baby and should not be thrown away, as it has antibodies which are protective.

5. **Early Childhood Care**

I. Do not allow a child's temperature to rise above 101 degree F because of any reason. It can cause febrile seizures
II. If a child gets a fit take him to doctor immediately.
III. Every child should be immunized against infectious diseases as per the recommended schedule of immunization.
IV. Do not allow a child to have too much contact with paint, newsprint ink, lead etc. as they are toxic.
V. Take precautions against head injury, and other accidents.
VI. Ensure that the child gets a well-balanced diet and clean drinking water.
VII. Introduce additional foods of good quality and in sufficient quantity when the child is 4 -6 months old.
VIII. Vitamin A deficiency and its consequences including night blindness can be easily prevented through the use of Vitamin A supplementation.
IX. Protect a child from Meningitis and Encephalitis by providing a hygienic environment which is free of overcrowding.
X. Common salt must be iodized as a precaution against goiter and cretinism.
XI. Do not allow a child to use hairpins, matchsticks and pencils, to remove wax from the ears.
XII. Use ear protectors to reduce the exposure to high levels of noise, if children are living or working in a noisy environment.
XIII. Do not slap a child over the face as this may lead to injury of the eardrum and consequent hearing loss

Locomotor disability

Disability of the bones, joint or muscles leading to substantial restriction of the movement of the limbs or a usual form of cerebral palsy. Some common conditions giving raise to locomotor disability could be poliomyelitis, cerebral palsy, amputation, injuries of spine, head, soft tissues, fractures, muscular dystrophies etc.

Blindness

A condition where a person suffers from any of the following conditions namely:

- Total absence of sight or
- Visual acuity not exceeding 6/60 or 20/200 (snellen) in the better eye with correcting lenses; or
- Limitation of the field vision subtending an angle of 20 degree or worse.

Person with low vision

A person with impairment of visual functioning even after treatment or standard refractive correction but who uses or is potentially capable of using vision for the planning or execution of a task with appropriate assistive device.

Hearing impairment

Loss of sixty decibels or more in the better ear in the conversational range of frequencies.

Mental illness

Any mental disorder other than mental retardation

- **Mental retardation** - A condition of arrested or incomplete development of mind of a person which is specially characterized by sub - normality of intelligence i.e. cognitive, language, motor and social abilities
- **Autism** - A condition of uneven skill development primarily affecting the communication and social abilities of a person, marked by repetitive and ritualistic behaviour.
- **Multiple Disability** - A combination of two or more disabilities as defined in clause (i) of section 2 of the Person with disabilities (Equal Opportunities, Protection of Rights and Full Participation) Act 1995 namely Blindness/low vision, Speech and Hearing Impairments, Locomotor disability including leprosy cured Mental retardation and Mental illness.

Learning Disabilities (Dyslexia)

Affect person's ability to acquire, process, and/or use either, spoken, read, written or nonverbal information(organization/planning, functional literacy skills, memory, reasoning, problem solving, perceptual skills) or in other words in short - difficulty with language in its various uses (not always reading).

- **Dyspraxia** - The inability to motor plan, to make an appropriate body response.
- **Dysgraphia** - Difficulty with the act of writing both in the technical as well as the expressive sense. There may also be difficulty with spelling.
- **Dyscalculia** - Difficulty with calculations.
- **Attention Deficit and Hyperactivity Disorder(ADHD)** - Hyperactivity, distractibility and impulsivity.

CHAPTER TWO

PHYSIOTHERAPEUTIC INTERVENTIONS

1. **EXERCISE THERAPY**

Exercise therapy is defined as a regimen or plan of physical activities designed and prescribed to facilitate the patients to recover from diseases and any conditions, which disturb their movement and activity of daily life or maintain a state of well-being [1] through neuro re-education, gait training, and therapeutic activities. It is systemic execution of planned physical movements, postures, or activities intended to enable the patients to (1) reduce risk, (2) enhance function, (3) remediate or prevent impairment, (4) optimize overall health, and (5) improve fitness and well-being [2].

This therapy may relate specific muscles or parts of the body, to general and strenuous activities that can return a recovering patient to the peak of physical condition. It is highly repetitive and intensive and requires time and dedication on the part of the patients to encourage neuroplasticity. The therapy is performed by professionals with an educational background in exercise physiology, exercise science, or other similar degree. To succeed goal-oriented treatment, the personnel must.

1. Provide comprehensive and personalized patient/individual management.
2. Implement a variety of therapeutic interventions that are complementary (e.g., heat application before joint mobilization and passive stretch, followed by active exercise to use new mobility in a functional manner).
3. Rely on clinical decision-making skill.

4. Promote patients' independence whenever possible through the use of home management,

Self-management exercise programs, and patient-related instruction.

In-house physical therapy by family, friends, or caregivers to deliver the appropriate exercise therapy in the home can greatly decrease healthcare costs which may limit the intervention.

Therefore, training and educating these persons are important in effective exercise therapy.

Exercise therapy can be called Activity-Based Therapy, Activity-Based Recovery Therapy,

Neuro-based Therapy and Restorative Therapy.

Objectives of exercise therapy

The objectives of exercise therapy are as following;

- Promote activity and minimize the effects of inactivity, increased independence
- Increase the normal range of motion.
- Improve strength the weak muscles.
- Improve the performance in daily activities.
- Enable ambulation.
- Release contracted muscles, tendons, and fascia.
- Improve circulation.
- Improve respiratory capacity.
- Improve coordination.
- Reduce rigidity.
- Improve balance.
- Promote relaxation.
- Increased motor or sensory function.
- Reduction of medication, reduction of hospital visits, and increased overall health.

The most important goal of exercise therapy is an optimal level of physical fitness by the end of the intervention. The physical fitness a state characterized by good muscle strength combined with good endurance.

Concept

Exercise therapy based on the independent movement which depends on individual goals.

It aims to improve the ability to achieve optimal daily functioning. To achieve the goal of exercise therapy, the practitioner needs to understand the disablement process which includes:

The disablement process

a) Impairment: A loss or abnormality of anatomic, physiologic, or psychologic structure or function.

b) Functional limitation: A limitation of the whole person performance, task in an efficient, typically expected, or competent manner, or a physical action activity.

c) Disability: The inability or a limitation to perform the performance of actions, or tasks.

Techniques

The techniques of exercise therapy used in treatment may be classified as follows.

- **Passive movements**

Passive movements (Motion Therapy, Continuous Passive) provide continuous passive motion to the applied joint. The apparatus can be used immediately after the operation to improve the range of motion, reduce pain, discomfort, and healing. This machine is adjustable, easily controlled, versatile, and usually electrically operated.

a) Relaxed passive movements
b) Accessory movements

Passive manual mobilization techniques
a) Mobilizations of joints
b) Manipulations of joints by
- Physiotherapists
- Surgeon/physician
c) Controlled sustained stretching of tightened structure:

- **Active exercise**

Movement performed or controlled by the voluntary action of muscles, working in opposition to an external force

Voluntary
a) Assisted active exercise
b) Free exercise

c) Assisted-resisted exercise
d) Resisted exercise

Exercise preparation

Before exercise training, a patient should be evaluated by a physician. It is important to exclude patients with ventricular hypertrophy, valvular heart disease, dangerous arrhythmias, and malignant hypertension. Other cardiac cases and patients at risk, such as those with exercise-induced asthma, obesity, or diabetes, should perform an exercise stress test under careful medical supervision. Blood pressure and heart rate and the electrocardiogram (ECG) must be monitored throughout the exercise to confirm their cardiovascular function.

- **Exercise for healthy individuals**

Continuously aerobic exercises that use large muscle groups are recommended including western and eastern style:

Western style
- Cycling
- Swimming
- Walking
- Running
- Jogging
- Aerobic dance/exercise classes
- Dancing
- Stair climbing
- Rowing
- Skating
- Jumping rope
- Cross-country skiing

Eastern style
- Tai chi
- Yoga
- Arm swing exercise
- Wand exercise

Equipment for Exercise therapy

There are many kinds of equipment for exercise therapy including:

- Hydrotherapy equipment

- Heat and cold therapy equipment (paraffin wax bath, moist heat therapy unit, moist heat therapy unit, stream/hot pack, infrared lamp).
- Treatment equipment (massage cum treatment table, tilt table, activity mattress, continuous passive motion unit, medicine ball, parallel bar, equilibrium board).
- Multi exercise therapy unit (complex exercising unit).
- Shoulder, arm, hand, leg, knee, foot exercise unit.
- Suspension unit.
- Mobility aids (Walkers, crutch, cane).
- Massage

Special techniques used in exercise therapy:

- *Frenkel's exercises* are used to treat the incoordination which results from many other diseases, for example, disseminated sclerosis
- *Proprioceptive neuromuscular facilitation* (PNF) is an approach in which treatment is directed at a total human being, not just at a specific problem or body segment.
- *Hydrotherapy* refers to the use of multi-depth immersion pools or tanks that facilitate the application of various established therapeutic interventions including stretching, joint mobilization, strengthening, etc.
- *Breathing exercises* are designed to retrain the muscles of respiration, improve ventilation, lessen the work of breathing, and improve gaseous exchange and patient's overall function in daily living activities.

2. ACTINOTHERAPY

It is generally carried on with quartz tubes containing vaporized mercury or with carbon arc lamps. Some hospitals use air-cooled mercury quartz apparatus; some have water-cooled equipment and *some* report using arc lamps A newer method of ultra-violet production is the cold quartz apparatus in which high frequency currents are used in a way similar to their use in the neon advertising signs.

The indications on which these forms of radiation therapy are prescribed are anemia, malnutrition, tuberculosis, pulmonary and extra-pulmonary; dermatologic conditions such as acne, psoriasis, erysipelas, cellulitis, carbuncles and furuncles. Various local conditions such as arthritis, infections, lumbago, myalgia, varicose ulcers, fractures, wounds, neuritis and sprains are favorite indications for radiation therapy, and actionotherapy is used extensively in bronchitis, coryza, pyorrhea and eye, ear, nose and throat conditions.

Equipments

- Outdoor sunlight
- Therapeutic lamps
- Deep therapy lamps
- Electric light baths
- Air-cooled ultra-violet
- Water-cooled ultra-violet
- Carbon arc lamp
- Infra-red
- Laser

Indications

- Dermatology
- Anaemia
- Tuberculosis
- Arthritis
- Tonic
- Infections
- Malnutrition
- Acne
- Neuritis
- Myalgia
- Eye, ear, nose and throat
- Bronchitis
- Varicose ulcer
- Fractures
- Sprains
- Furuncles
- Carbuncles
- Lumbago
- Rheumatism
- Coryza
- Psoriasis

- Myositis
- Wounds
- Dental
- Neuralgia
- Obesity

3. HYDROTHERAPY

Hydrotherapy (Aqua-therapy) is any activity performed in water to assist in rehabilitation and recovery from e.g. hard training or serious injury. It is a form of exercise in warm water and is a popular treatment for patients with neurologic and musculoskeletal conditions. The goals of this therapy are muscle relaxation, improving joint motion and reducing pain.

Physical properties of water

In common with other forms of matter, water has certain physical properties which include mass, weight, density, relative density, buoyancy, hydrostatic pressure, surface tension, refraction and reflection.

Of the physical laws of water that the physiotherapist should understand and apply when giving Aquatherapy, those of buoyancy and hydrostatic pressure are the most important. The lateral pressure exerted and the effect of buoyancy together will give the feeling of weightlessness.

Physiological effects

The physiological effects of water therapy combine those brought by the hot water of the pool with those of the exercises. The extent of the effects varies with the temperature of the water, the length of the treatment and the type and severity of the exercise. The physiological effects of exercise in water are similar to those of exercise on dry land. The blood supply to the working muscles is increased, heat is evolved with each chemical change occurring during the contraction, and the muscles temperature rises. There is an increased metabolism in the muscles resulting in a greater demand for oxygen and increased production of carbon dioxide. These changes augment the similar changes brought about by the heat of the water, and both contribute towards the final effect. The range of joint movement is either maintained or increased, and muscle power increases. During the immersion the physiological effects are similar to those brought about by any other form of heat but less localized. A rise in body temperature is inevitable because the body gains heat from the water and from all the contracting muscles performing the exercises. As the skin becomes heated the superficial blood vessels dilate and the peripheral blood supply is increased. The blood flowing through these vessels is heated and by convection, the temperature of the underlying structures rises.

The relatively mild heat of the water reduces the sensitivity of sensory nerve endings and the muscle tone will diminish when the muscles are warmed by the blood passing through them.

Therapeutic effects

- Relieve pain and muscle spasm
- To gain relaxation
- To maintain or increase the range of joint movement
- To re-educate paralyzed muscles
- To strengthen weak muscles and to develop their power and endurance.
- To encourage walking and other functional and recreational activities.
- To improve circulation (tropic condition of the skin)
- To give the patient encouragement and confidence in carrying out his exercises, thereby improving his morale.
- The warmth of water blocks nociception by acting on thermal receptors and mechanoreceptors, thus influencing spinal segmental mechanisms.
- Warm water stimulates blood flow positively, which leads to muscle relaxation.
- The hydrostatic effect may relieve pain by reducing peripheral edema and by dampening the sympatic nervous system activity.

Clinical Contraindications

- Cardiovascular disease
- Cardiopulmonary disease
- Diabetic
- Balance disorder
- History of CVA, Epilepsy
- Incontinence
- Labyrinthitis
- a cold
- Influenza
- Fever
- Skin conditions
- Chemical allergies (Chlorine)

- Contagious diseases
- Hepatitis
- Tracheotomy
- Urinary tract infection
- Serious Epilepsy
- Urinary incontinence
- Open Wounds
- Recently Surgery
- Hydrophobic

Aquatic Therapy in Sports

- Aquatic exercise refers to the use of water that facilitates the application of established therapeutic interventions, including stretching, strengthening, jt mobilization, balance, gait training and endurance training.
- Aquatic therapy is beneficial in the management of patients with musculoskeletal problems, neurologic problems, cardiopulmonary pathology, and other conditions.
- Aquatic therapy has rapidly become a popular rehabilitation technique among athletic trainers.
- It is gaining acceptance to facilitate overall fitness, cross-training, and sport-specific skills.
- Aquatic therapy is believed to be beneficial because it increases joint compression forces.
- The perception of weightlessness experienced in the water seems to decrease muscular pain and spasm that can carry over into the patient's daily functional activities.
- The primary goal of aquatic therapy is to teach the athlete how to use water as a modality for improving movement, strength, and fitness.

Goals and Indications

- To facilitate functional recovery.
- Facilitate ROM exercises.
- Initiates resistance training.
- Facilitate weight-bearing activities.
- Enhance delivery of manual techniques.

- Provide **3-D** access to the patients.
- Facilitate cardiovascular exercise.
- Initiate functional activity replication.
- Minimize risk to injury or reinjures during rehabilitation
- Enhance patient's relaxation
- The program must also be specific and individualized to the athlete's particular injury and sports if it is to be successful.

Physical Property of Water

- Buoyancy
- Density & Specific Gravity
- Hydrostatic Pressure
- Viscosity
- Resistive force and
- Thermodynamics.
- The trainer must understand several physical properties of the water before designing a aquatic therapy program.

Buoyancy

- One of the primary forces involved in aquatic therapy.
- It is the upward force that works opposite to gravity.
- Archimedes principle states that an immersed body experiences upward thrust equal to the volume of liquid displaced.
- Because of this buoyant force, a person entering the water experiences an apparent loss of wt.
- Buoyancy can be determined by several factors like the ratio of bone weight to muscle weight, the amount and distribution of fat and the depth and expansion of the chest.

Density & Specific Gravity

- Any object with a specific gravity less than that of water will float.
- Specific gravity of all body parts is not uniform.
- On the average, humans have slightly lesser density and specific gravity(0.974) than water, with men averaging higher density than

women.
- Lean body mass, which includes bone, muscle, connective tissue, and organs, have a typical density near 1.1, whereas fat mass, which includes both essential body fat plus fat in excess of essential needs, has a density of about 0.9.
- Highly fit and muscular men tend toward specific gravities greater than one, whereas an unfit or obese man might be considerably less.
- The lungs, when filled with air, the specific gravity of the chest area decreases. This allows the head and chest to float higher in the water than the heavier, denser extremities.

Hydrostatic Pressure

- It is the Pressure exerted by the water on immersed objects.
- Pascal's law states that the pressure exerted by fluid on an immersed object is equal on all surfaces of the body.
- Hydrostatic pressure is directly proportional to the density of water and depth of the immersion of objects.
- Blood displaces cephalic (assists venous return), right atrial pressure begins to rise (centralizes peripheral blood flow), pleural surface pressure rises, the chest wall compresses, and the diaphragm is displaced cephalic.

Viscosity

- Viscosity refers to the magnitude of internal friction specific to a fluid during motion resulting in resistance to flow.
- Resistance from viscosity is proportional to the velocity of movement through liquid.
- A limb moving relative to water is subjected to the resistive effects of the fluid called drag force and turbulence when present. Under turbulent flow conditions, this resistance increases as a log function of velocity.

Resistive force

1. Cohesive force: Runs parallel to the water surface. Closely related to surface tension.

2. Bow force: Generated in front of the object during movement. Increase in the front but decrease in the rear pressure of the moving object.
3. Drag force: It is a backward force formed by the Eddies in the low pressure zone.

Thermodynamics

- Water is an efficient conductor, transferring heat 25 times faster than air.
- Water may be used therapeutically over a wide range of temp.
- Cold plunge tanks are often used in athletic training at temp of 10°–15°C to produce a decrease in muscle pain and speed recovery from overuse injury.
- Typically, therapy pools operate in the range of 33.5°–35.5°C, temp that permit lengthy immersion durations and exercise activities sufficient to produce therapeutic effects without chilling or overheating.
- Hot tubs are usually maintained at 37.5°– 41°C.
- Heat transfer begins immediately on immersion, and as the heat capacity of the human body is less than that of water, the body equilibrates faster than water does.

Studies have shown that aquatic exercise requires a higher energy expenditure than the same exercise performed on land.

- It is an effective means of alternate fitness training (cross-training) for the injured athlete.
- It should be noted that a study of shallow water running (xiphoid level) and deep-water running (using an aqua jogger), at the same rate of perceived exertion found a significant difference of 10 beats/min in heart rate, with shallow-water running demonstrating a greater heart rate.
- The athlete can maintain a near normal maximal aerobic capacity with aquatic exercise.
- A/C to a study, for maintenance of cardio respiratory conditioning in highly fit individuals, water running in respect to dry land running is effective for the maintenance of maximum VO2 when training intensities and frequencies duration are same.

Contraindications

- Infections, fever, temp.
- Open wounds, surgical incisions.
- Contagious skin diseases.
- Seizures.
- Serious cardiac conditions.
- Hydrophobia.
- Allergy to pool chemicals.

Precautions

- Recently healed wound or incision.
- Altered peripheral sensation.
- Asthma.
- Seizures controlled with medications.
- Fear of water.

Disadvantages

- Costly and maintenance is high.
- Inadequately trained therapists.
- Stabilization in water is more difficult than that on land.
- Thermoregulation issues with the athletes as the temp cannot be controlled.
- Shivering in water.
- Tolerance to heat on land cannot be maintained after aquatic therapy.

Equipments

- Collars, Rings, Belts, and vests.
- Swim bars.
- Gloves, Hand paddles, and Hydro-tone balls.
- Fins and hydro-tone boots.
- Kickboards.
- Floats.
- Masks.
- Pool toys.
- Pool with treadmill.

Components

- Warm-up
- Strengthening / mobility activities
- Endurance/ cardiovascular activities
- Stretching/ cool down

Upper extremity

- Chest deep water allows scapular and thoracic support.
- Walking front, back and sideways, natural arm swing constitutes warm up.
- Generally treatment is given in supine and prone.
- The athlete will need flotation equipment for cervical, lumbar and lower extremity support in order to have upper extremity exercises.
- For Stretching, mobilization and ROM exercises.
- Progression in strength training done with the use of dumbbells.
- Progressive resistive exercises.
- PNF
- Functional training

Spine

- Unloading nature of water exercises relieves spine dysfunctions.
- For total body balance and neuromuscular control.
- Trunk stabilization against anterior and posterior forces/oblique and diagonal forces.
- Tuck and roll exercise.
- The athlete's ability of stability using deep-water activities in vertical position while bringing knees to chest and progressing to tucking and rolling type movements.

Lower extremities

- Running forward and backwards against tubing resistance.
- Supported single lower extremity running movement.
- Supine alternating hip knee flexion extension, progress to single-leg reverse squats.

- Progress from NWB to WB.
- Initially athlete may need assistance with flotation but progressively decreases the amount of flotation.
- For the athlete, the deep water allows for a workout along with maintaining strength in uninvolved joints.
- Activities can involve running, bicycling, cross training etc.
- For progression, floatation cuffs can be used.
- Practice can be done by standing on uneven surface like noddle or kickboard.

4. ELECTROTHERAPY

Electrotherapy is the use of electrical energy as a medical treatment. In medicine, the term *electrotherapy* can apply to a variety of treatments, including the use of electrical devices such as deep brain stimulators for neurological disease. The term has also been applied specifically to the use of electric current to speed wound healing. Additionally, the term "electrotherapy" or "electromagnetic therapy" has also been applied to a range of alternative medical devices and treatments.

Methods

- Electrical Stimulation
- Transcutaneous Electrical Nerve Stimulation (TENS)
- Infra Red Irradiation (IRR)
- Ultrasound
- Interferential Therapy (IFT)
- Shortwave Diathermy (SWD)
- Low Intensity Pulsed Ultrasound (LIPUS)
- Neuromuscular Electrical Stimulation (NMES)
- Microwave Diathermy (MWD)
- Shortwave Therapy (PSWT)
- Functional Electrical Stimulation (FES)
- Laser Therapy
- Faradic Stimulation
- Hydrocollator Packs
- Microwave Therapy
- Iontophoresis
- Wax Therapy

- Low Intensity RF Applications
- High Voltage Pulsed Galvanic Stimulation (HVPGS)
- Balneotherapy (inc spa/whirlpool)
- Pulsed Electromagnetic Fields (PEMF's)
- Low Intensity Direct Current (LIDC) and Pulsed LIDC
- Fluidotherapy
- Microcurrent Therapies
- Twin Peak Monophasic Stimulation
- Therapeutic Ultrasound
- Diadynamic Therapy
- Pulsed Magnetic Therapy
- Static Magnetic Therapy
- Russian Stimulation
- Microcurrent Therapy

Uses of Electrotherapy
1. Pain management
2. Treatment of neuromuscular dysfunction
3. Improves range of joint mobility
4. Tissue repair
5. Acute and chronic edema
6. Peripheral blood flow
7. Iontophoresis
8. Urine and fecal incontinence
9. Lymphatic Drainage

Effectiveness for particular indications

- Musculoskeletal conditions
- Neck and back pain
- Shoulder disorders
- Other musculoskeletal disorders
- Chronic pain
- Chronic wounds

5. **MANUAL THERAPY**

   Definition:

According the *American Academy of Orthopaedic Manual Physical Therapists (AAOMPT)* orthopaedic manual physical therapy (OMPT) is defined as:

"OMPT is any "hands-on" treatment provided by the physical therapist. Treatment may include moving joints in specific directions and at different speeds to regain movement (joint mobilization and manipulation), muscle stretching, passive movements of the affected body part, or having the patient move the body part against the therapist's resistance to improve muscle activation and timing. Selected specific soft tissue techniques may also be used to improve the mobility and function of tissue and muscles."

The International Federation of Orthopaedic Manipulative Physical Therapists (IFOMPT) defines manual therapy techniques as:

"Skilled hand movements intended to produce any or all of the following effects: improve tissue extensibility; increase range of motion of the joint complex; mobilize or manipulate soft tissues and joints; induce relaxation; change muscle function; modulate pain; and reduce soft tissue swelling, inflammation or movement restriction."

Terminology

The International Federation of Orthopaedic Manipulative Physical Therapists (IFOMPT) has offered the following definitions:

Manipulation: A passive, high velocity, low amplitude thrust applied to a joint complex within its anatomical limit with the intent to restore optimal motion, function, and/ or to reduce pain.

Mobilization: A manual therapy technique comprising a continuum of skilled passive movements to the joint complex that are applied at varying speeds and amplitudes, that may include a small-amplitude/high velocity therapeutic movement (manipulation) with the intent to restore optimal motion, function, and/ or to reduce pain.

The American Academy of Orthopaedic Manual Physical Therapists (AAOMPT) has proposed the following framework for describing manipulative interventions :

1. **Rate of force application**: Describe the rate at which the force was applied.

2. **Location in range of available movement**: Describe whether motion was intended to occur only at the beginning, towards the middle, or at the end point of the available range of movement. The term available range of movement is intended to describe the available movement as perceived by the therapist after the patient has been positioned and at the time the

technique is applied. The available movement may or may not be the same as the range of motion available at a particular joint or region under other circumstances.

3. **Direction of force**: Describe the direction in which the therapist imparts the force. This description should be devoid of the "intent" of the technique and, instead, should follow standard anatomical and biomechanical conventions.

4. **Target of force**: Describe the location where the therapist intended to apply the force. In the case of the spine, force may be directed at a specific level, or more generally across a particular region such as mid lumbar or lower thoracic.

5. **Relative structural movement**: Describe which structure or region was intended to remain stable and which structure or region was intended to move, naming the moving structure or region first and the stable segment second, separated by the word "on." For example, a "lower lumbar on upper lumbar" technique implies that the clinician intended to move the lower lumbar region while stabilizing the upper lumbar region. Techniques associated with the peripheral joints would be described utilizing the same convention (eg, tibia on femur, humerus on scapular glenoid).

6. **Patient position**: Describe the position of the patient (eg, supine, prone, recumbent). This would include any premanipulative positioning of a region of the body, such as being positioned in rotation or side bending.

Mobilization and Manipulation Techniques

- Elbow Mobilizations
- Wrist/Hand Mobilizations
- Hip Mobilizations
- Knee Mobilizations
- Ankle/Foot Mobilizations
- Spinal_Manipulation
- Shoulder Mobilizations and Manipulation
- Cervicothoracic Manipulation

CHAPTER THREE

THERAPEUTIC APPROACHES IN VARIOUS CONDITIONS

1. *PHYSIOTHERAPY IN NEUROLOGICAL CONDITIONS*

The term 'neurological conditions' comprises a wide range of diseases and injuries that affect the central and/or peripheral nervous system. It is however possible to subcategorize neurological conditions. Presented below is an overview of the types of physiotherapy treatment that patients with neurological conditions benefit from.

Physiotherapy for Degenerative Neurological Conditions

Two examples of degenerative neurological conditions are Multiple Sclerosis (MS) and Amyotrophic Lateral Sclerosis (ALS). These are diseases that degrade the function of the neurological system over time. Little can be done to stop the progression of these types of diseases but Physiotherapists can still have a profoundly positive effect of the quality of life of patients living with these diseases.

Physiotherapy for degenerative neurological conditions is focused on:

- Strategies to compensate for any lost neurological function
- Exercises to preserve function that remains
- Preservation of the patient's joint mobility and strength
- Preservation of balance
- Preservation of activities of daily living (such as dressing, cooking, cleaning etc)
- Prescribing devices to aid with tasks that have become difficult

- Prescribing mobility aids
- Education on their condition
- Evaluation of the progression of their condition

Physiotherapy Secondary Neurological Conditions

A secondary neurological condition can be defined as one that has developed as a result of some other pathological process. Two examples of this are Stroke, which develops as a result of an event limiting blood flow to part of the brain and the neurological impairment that can result from a mass or tumor in the brain. The symptoms and impact of these conditions depends entirely on what part of the brain is affected and how widespread the damage is. Recovery after stroke or after the successful treatment of a brain tumor is possible owing to the amazing ability of the brain to adapt and reorganize itself called neural plasticity.

Physiotherapy for secondary neurological conditions is focused on stimulating neurological plasticity so that the patient can regain functions that they have lost. Because of this, treatment plans vary widely and are designed to address the specific deficits that the patient is experiencing. Neurological Physiotherapists must be creative individuals who can devise complex treatment plans with tasks that progress toward the patients goals.

Physiotherapy for Traumatic Neurological Conditions

Neurological impairments can also be the result of trauma. Some examples are head injuries/concussions, spinal cord injuries or peripheral nerve injuries resulting from a traumatic event. These are very specialized areas of Physiotherapy that require specific training and expertise. Physiotherapy is very successful at helping people with these types of injuries recover and to live more full and normal lives. A complete recovery is not possible for all people with neurological impairments. However, the vast majority can be helped a great deal by a Physiotherapist skilled in Neurological rehabilitation.

Neurological disorders are among the most challenging diagnoses to have for both the patient and the Physiotherapist. However, the impact that Physiotherapy has on the lives of people with Neurological impairments in enormous.

2. *PHYSIOTHERAPY IN PAEDIATRIC CONDITIONS*

Paediatric physiotherapists work with people of varying ages from premature babies to adolescents to ensure optimal physical function and development. Like all physiotherapists, they are concerned with movement, co-ordination, posture and the cardio-respiratory system. The aim of the paediatric physiotherapist is to provide a program that the client will enjoy, while encouraging them to participate and become independent.

Paediatric physiotherapists aim to minimise the effects of physical impairment to promote optimum function and musculoskeletal development. Advice on activities and stretches offered by the physiotherapist can assist in maintaining full range of movement and prevention of contracture.

Paediatric physiotherapists assess and treat infants and children with a range of conditions including:

- cerebral palsy - from mild hemiplegia to severe quadriplegia;
- developmental delay - due to hypotonia with or without diagnosis and may be gross motor or global;and other genetic conditions;
- spina bifida and neural tube defects;
- muscular dystrophy and spinal muscular atrophy;
- brachial plexus lesions;
- juvenile chronic arthritis (JCA);
- visual handicaps;
- premature babies with dystonia;
- postural problems - torticollis, scoliosis, talipes, metatarsus adductus, or idiopathic toe walkers;
- respiratory problems such as cystic fibrosis or asthma;
- osteogenis imperfecta;
- minimal cerebral dysfunction

The role of the paediatric physiotherapist is to assess the referred child and give parents and/or carers advice regarding handling, positioning and treatment through play and/or exercise. Physiotherapists work closely with families, carers, teachers, doctors and other health professionals. The approach is holistic and practical, with an emphasis on gross motor function and posture. For better outcomes and most effective treatment results, early referral is the key (before eight months). Infants and children can be seen at home, day care centre, Early Intervention Programs, schools or clinics on a regular basis.

Advice will be given on appropriate handling and equipment including seating, standing frames, mobility aids and pushers. A range of treatment methods may be used such as neuro-developmental therapy, motor learning and hydrotherapy. Physiotherapists are often the first therapist to see the child and are well received by parents.

Paediatric physiotherapists also work with a range of conditions to help older children and adolescents, including:

- acquired brain injury and spinal injury;
- neurological diseases
- post trauma injuries, such as fractures, sports injuries, post orthopaedic surgery;
- juvenile chronic arthritis and related conditions;
- developmental conditions such as cerebral palsy, muscular dystrophy and spina bifida;
- cystic fibrosis and other respiratory disorders such as asthma;
- burns and plastic surgery;
- limb deficiency conditions;
- chronic pain

Physiotherapists help to maintain and develop functional skill level and range of movement in order to minimise joint contracture and postural deformities. They encourage children to partake in a wide range of activities at school and in the community to maintain physical fitness and provide opportunities for socialisation with their peers. They also prescribe and monitor the use of aids such as orthotics, walking aids, and wheelchairs to help maintain independence.

3. *PHYSIOTHERAPY IN ORTHOPAEDICS CONDITIONS*

Orthopaedics relates to the branch of medicine and surgery concerned with the diseases, conditions and injuries of the musculoskeletal system, namely bones, joints, soft tissues (muscles, tendon, and ligaments) and neural tissue.

A major aspect of the role of physiotherapy in orthopedics is to rehabilitate after trauma, most commonly bone fractures and joint dislocations. Depending on the nature and extent of the damage sustained, some patients will have undergone surgery followed by a period of immobilisation in a cast or splint, whilst others are treated by immobilisation only. This provides a stable environment for optimal healing to occur. However, once healing is complete and the referral to physiotherapy has been made, the challenging process of rehabilitation has to commence. This includes the regaining of normal joint movement, full strength, co-ordination, balance and function. Physiotherapists' role is also to provide advice and guidance regarding the return to work, driving, and sport and leisure activities.

Physiotherapy role in rehabilitate to some of the fallowing orthopaedics conditions:

- Pre and Post Surgical Care of all Orthopaedic Conditions
- Balance/Vertigo Rehabilitation
- Postural Training
- Arthritis Management
- Back/Neck Rehabilitation
- Joint Pain Management
- Spinal Stabilization
- Muscle and Ligament Strains and Sprains
- Myofascial Release
- Road trafic Accident Injuries
- Work Injuries

The most common orthopaedic conditions that many patients present to our practices with include post-fracture, osteopenia, osteoporosis and osteoarthritis.

Osteopenia is a condition characterised by less than normal bone density and can increase an individual's risk of developing osteoporosis.

Osteoporosis is a systemic skeletal disease that is associated with low bone mass, deterioration of bone tissue and compromised bone strength. As a consequence, this leads to an increase in bone fragility and susceptibility to fracture, particularly of the wrist, hip and spine. Whilst the role of the physiotherapist in dealing with the consequences of osteoporosis, in terms of the rehabilitation after an osteoporotic fracture may be obvious, our preventative or prophylactic role is of equal importance. It is widely accepted that participation in suitable weight-bearing exercise can reduce the risk of development of osteoporosis, although other factors including normal hormone levels and sufficient calorific intake (especially protein) and adequate levels of calcium and vitamin D are required to achieve adequate peak bone mass. Physiotherapists are therefore expertly positioned to give advice and education regarding the most appropriate form of weight-bearing exercise to be undertaken for an individual with osteoporosis, taking age, gender, and general physical condition into account. Other important aspects of physiotherapy intervention in osteoporosis can include pain management if this is a feature and the prevention of falls by implementing balance re-education and strengthening programmes.

Osteoarthritis (OA) or mechanical arthritis is another common orthopaedic condition. It is characterised by the degeneration of joints due to the breakdown of joint cartilage. When the bony surfaces of a joint become less well protected by cartilage as a result of degeneration, the underlying bone may become exposed and damaged. These degenerative changes usually result in bone and joint inflammation and the development of pain, swelling, stiffness, locking and clicking with in the affected joint. In the acute phase, physiotherapy treatment is primarily aimed at symptom resolution and minimisation and to restore normal movement, strength and function. The emphasis then switches towards facilitating self-directed management by dispensing practical advice and prescribing appropriate individual home exercise programmes to keep exacerbations of the underlying condition to an absolute minimum.

Inflammatory arthropathies such as rheumatoid arthritis (RA), septic arthritis, gout, juvenile idiopathic arthritis and spondylarthropathies (ankylosing spondylitis, reactive arthritis and psoriatic arthropathy)

Soft tissue disorders such as low back pain, tennis elbow, golfer's elbow etc.

Physiotherapy treatment has a vital role to play. Following a thorough musculoskeletal assessment, a goal-oriented treatment plan may include the following:

- Pain management, via the application of heat, ice and electrotherapeutic modalities,

- Joint protection, through the prescription of splints and supports if indicated (and often in conjunction with occupational therapy colleagues)

- Prevention of deformities, by means of joint range of movement exercises, stretches to improve flexibility and advice regarding good posture

- Rehabilitation and the regaining of function via strengthening and conditioning programmes and gait re-education etc.

The neck and back areas are comprised of various complexes structures, which add to the complexity of these conditions. The vertebrae, which form the bony structure of the spine, protect the spinal cord. The joints between the vertebrae and their supporting ligaments, muscles and tendons allow multi-directional movement. The discs in between the vertebrae act as shock absorbers and further facilitate movement. Therefore correct identification of the tissue or structure that is causing the problem and accurate diagnosis is essential to ensure that the most effective treatment plan is put in place. Following the assessment process, the physiotherapy treatment for back and neck problems may include:

- Manual joint mobilisations
- Spinal manipulations
- Mechanical or manual traction
- Electrotherapy modalities
- Trigger point dry needling
- Soft tissue techniques
- Prophylactic management (postural and ergonomic advice, manual handling instruction, flexibility and core musculature conditioning programmes, back care advice and self management).

The common causes of neck and back pain can include strains of the joints between the vertebra due to ligament strain, muscular strains and spasms, disc lesions including bulges and herniations/prolapses, sciatica arising from pressure on or irritation of the sciatic nerve roots by a disc lesion, poor posture, degenerative changes of the joints or discs due to general 'wear and tear', traumatic injuries such as whiplash or vertebral fractures, and acquired conditions and diseases such as osteoarthritis, rheumatological conditions (such as Rheumatoid Arthitis and Ankylosing Spondylitis), osteoporosis and structural problems such as scoliosis (a sideways curvature of the spine). Physiotherapy intervention, through a combination of reducing pain and improving movement and strength, can significantly improve function and thus quality of life. Patients can more effectively manage their condition, continue to remain active and minimise the effect on their everyday life.

Physiotherapy can play a vital role in the effectiveness of orthopaedic surgery and in many cases can influence the outcome. Whilst the repair of damaged structures is accomplished during surgery, the rehabilitation process is extremely important to ensure that healing is complete and that full function is recovered. The most common surgical procedures that we provide treatment and rehabilitation programmes for include the following:

Hip Surgery – arthroscopy, repair of labral tears and CAM lesions (femoro-acetabular impingement), open reduction and internal fixation (surgical repair of fractures), resurfacing and total hip replacement surgery.

Knee Surgery – arthroscopy, repair of meniscal (cartilage) tears, cruciate ligament reconstruction, micro-fracturing, partial and total knee replacement surgery.

Ankle and Foot Surgery – open reduction and internal fixation (surgical repair of fractures), bunionectomy, tendon repairs, ankle stabilisation surgery.

Shoulder Surgery – arthroscopy, bursectomy, acromioplasty, rotator cuff tendon repairs, partial and total shoulder replacement surgery.

Spinal Surgery – microdiscectomy, laminectomy, foraminectomy, stabilisation of vertebral fractures.

Whilst it is not possible to reverse the degeneration and erosion of the joint cartilage and underlying bone, Physiotherapy can help reduce the symptoms caused by these processes. Weakness and wasting of the muscles adjacent to and surrounding the affected joints can be addressed by the prescription of specific strengthening exercises. Supportive splints, braces and orthoses may also be of benefit, for example prescription insoles can provide support and shock absorption to reduce pain associated with OA of the joints of the foot. Others prefer to adopt a maintenance approach to their treatment, and present at regular infrequent intervals, even when they are asymptomatic. This allows us to evaluate their progress with their home exercise regime, but also to pre-empt and 'trouble-shoot' problems and thus prevent severe exacerbations from developing.

Education is also an integral part of physiotherapy management in rheumatological conditions to assist the patient to self manage their condition in the longer term. In more severe cases, a multi-disciplinary approach is indicated, to promote independence and enable the patient to achieve and maintain their optimum potential at home, work and in social situations.

4. *PHYSIOTHERAPY IN CARDIOTHORACIC CONDITIONS*

Cardiovascular disease (CVD) refers to a group of conditions involving the heart, blood vessels, or the sequelae of poor blood supply due to a diseased vascular supply. Over 82% of the mortality burden is caused by ischaemic or coronary heart disease (IHD), stroke (both haemorrhagic and ischaemic), hypertensive heart disease or congestive heart failure (CHF). Over the past decade, CVD has become the single largest cause of death worldwide, representing nearly 30% of all deaths and about 50% of NCD deaths. In 2016, CVD caused an estimated 17.9 million deaths, representing 31% of all deaths worldwide. Behavioural risk factors such as physical inactivity, tobacco use and unhealthy diet explain nearly 80% of the CVD burden.

What are cardiovascular diseases?

CVDs include a wide range of conditions, such as the following:

Coronary Heart Disease (CHD), Cerebrovascular Disease, Peripheral Arterial Disease (/Peripheral_Arterial_Disease), Rheumatic Heart Disease, Congenital Heart Disease, Deep Vein Thrombosis (DVT), Pulmonary Embolism.

85% of CVD deaths are due to heart attacks and strokes. These are generally acute events caused by blockage, preventing blood flow to the heart or brain. The most common cause for these blockages is due to a process called atherosclerosis.

Who is at risk?

Modifiable risk factors of CVD include

- unhealthy diet
- physical inactivity
- smoking
- increased consumption of alcohol

Individuals with such behaviours may present with increased blood pressure, lipids and glucose levels, as well as being overweight or obese.

Non-Modifiable risk factors include

- Family history
- Age
- Gender - men at greater risk than pre-menopausal women; post menopausal women are at similar risk as men
- Ethnicity
- Socioeconomic status

Symptoms of CVD

Often the first warning of an underlying cardiovascular disease is a heart attack or stroke.

Symptoms of a heart attack may include:

- pain or discomfort in centre of chest
- Pain or discomfort in arms, left shoulder, elbows, jaw, or back.
- Shortness of breath
- Nausea or vomiting
- Light-headedness
- Pallor
- Cold *sweat*

Symptoms of a stroke may include the following:.

- unilateral weakness of face, arms or legs
- confusion, difficulty speaking or understanding speech
- dizziness
- difficulty seeing with one or both eyes
- headache
- fainting

How Physiotherapists Can Help?

Cardiac rehab programmes have been shown to be very effective, with physiotherapists playing a key role in these programmes. They have been shown to reduce length of hospital stay as well as number of cardiovascular related admissions, cardiac mortality and improved quality of life. Cardiac rehab classes include exercise, education and support. Physical activity performed at an intensity of >40% of maximal aerobic capacity has shown the greatest benefits in reducing the development or progressing of CVD. For every one metabolic equivalent (MET) increase in aerobic fitness there is a reduction of 8-17% in premature death. Aerobic exercise increases people's cardiac output, maximum heart rate, endurance, and arterial blood flow. It may also enhance their blood lipid profiles. For people who already have cardiovascular disease, prescribed aerobic exercise programs by physiotherapists can reduce their risk long-term. Aerobic conditioning activities such as running, rowing and walking along with resistance strength training exercises have been shown to be inversely associated with the risk of coronary heart disease.

Phases of Cardiac Rehabilitation (CR)

Cardiac rehabilitation typically comprises of four phases. The term phase is used to describe the varying time frames following a cardiac event. The secondary prevention component of CR requires delivery of exercise training, education and counselling, risk factor intervention and follows up.

Phase I: In hospital patient period

2-5 days

Member of Cardiac Rehab team (CRT) should visit the patient to;

- Give support and information to them and their families regarding heart disease
- Assist the patient to identify personal CV risk factors
- Discuss lifestyle modifications of personal risk factors and help provide an individual plan to support these lifestyle changes
- Gain support from family members to assist the patient in maintaining the necessary progress
- Plan a personal discharge activity programme and encourage the patient to adhere to this and commence daily walks
- Inform patients regarding phase II and phase III programs if available and encourage their attendance

At this stage emphasis is on counteracting the negative effects of a cardiac event not promoting training adaptations. Activity levels should be progressed using a staged approach which should be based on the patient's medical condition. Patient should be closely monitored for any signs of cardiac decompensation. Educational sessions should be commenced providing information regarding: The cardiac event, Psychological reactions to the event, Cardiac pain/symptom management, Correction of cardiac misconceptions.

Phase II: Post discharge period
Goals:

- Reinforce cardiac risk factor modification
- Provide education and support to patient and family
- Promote continuing adherence to lifestyle recommendations.

Support and education can be provided through

- Home visits
- Phone calls
- Outpatient reviews

Phase III: Cardiac Rehabilitation and secondary prevention
Structured exercise training with continual educational and psychological support and advice on risk factors. Should take a menu based approach and be individually tailored. Typically lasts at least 6 weeks with patients exercising 2/7 minimum. Exercise class will consist of warm up, exercise class, cool down – may also include resistance training with active recovery stations where appropriate.

Phase III compromises of all the following;

- Exercise prescription based on Clinical status
- Risk Stratification
- Previous activity
- Future needs

Education for patient and family regarding:

- Cardiac anatomy and physiology
- Recognition of cardiac pain and symptom management
- Risk factor identification and management
- Benefits of Physical Activities
- Energy conservation techniques/graded return to ADLs
- Cardio protective healthy eating

- Benefits and entitlements
- Stress management and relaxation techniques
- Counselling and behaviour modification
- Smoking cessation
- Vocational counselling

Sample format of a cardiac rehabilitation class
1. Check in (vitals assessed)
2. Warm Up (15 mins)
3. Main class (30 mins)
4. Cool down (10 mins)
5. Monitoring and reassessment of vitals and check out

1. **Warm Up**

Purpose: Prepare the body for exercise by raising the pulse rate in a graduated and safe way
Effects:

- redistributes blood to active tissues
- increases muscle temperature and speed of muscle action and relaxation
- prepares the mind
- prepares the muscle for the ROM involved for the conditioning period

Should include pulse raising activities (5 minutes) e.g. Marching on the spot, walking, low level cycle followed by stretching of the major muscle groups (5 mins) followed by more pulse raising activity.
NB: should try to keep feet moving at all times to maintain HR and body temp and avoid pooling.

2. **Main Class**

- For group rehab circuit training seems most popular. Depending on CV status and functional capacity patients may adopt an interval or continuous approach to the circuit.
- Separate stations are set out and participants spend a fixed amount of time at each aerobic station (30secs-2mins) before moving onto the next station which may be rest or active recovery in the form of resistance

work targeted at specific muscle groups.
- Resistance work as set out by ACSM 2006 – 10-15 reps to moderate fatigue of 8-10 exercises. Individualisation of the CV component can be achieved by varying; duration spent at each CV station, intensity (increase resistance, speed or ROM), period of rest, overall duration of the class.

3. **Cool Down**

   10 minutes at the end
   Goal: bring the body back to its resting state
   Should incorporate movements of diminishing intensity and passive stretching of the major muscle groups.
   Necessary because of;

- Increased risk of hypotension
- Older hearts take longer to return to resting levels
- Raised sympathetic activity during exercise increases the risk of arrhythmias immediately post exercise.

Phase IV: Maintenance

Goal: facilitate long term maintenance of lifestyle changes, monitoring risk factor changes and secondary prevention.
Options:

- Educational sessions
- Support groups
- Telephone follow up
- Review in clinics
- Outreach programmes
- Phase IV exercise programme organised by qualified phase IV gym instructor
- Links with GP and primary health care team
- Ongoing involvement of partners/spouses/family

Health and Safety

- Patient shouldn't exercise if they are generally unwell, symptomatic or clinically unstable on arrival;
- Fever/acute systemic illness
- Unresolved/unstable angina
- Resting BP systolic >200mmHg and diastolic > 110mmHg
- Significant drop in BP
- Symptomatic hypotension
- Resting/uncontrolled tachycardia (>100bpm)
- Uncontrolled atrial or ventricular arrhythmias
- New/recurrent symptoms of breathlessness, lethargy, palpitations, dizziness
- Unstable heart failure
- Unstable/uncontrolled diabetes

Need to consider the following;

- Local written policy clearly displayed for the management of emergency situations
- Rapid access to emergency team in hospital or via ambulance
- Regular checking and maintenance of all equipment
- Drinking water and glucose supplements available as required
- Access to and from venue, emergency exits, toilets and changing areas, lighting, surface and room space checked to ensure they're appropriate
- Enough space for patient traffic and safe placement of equipment
- Adequate temperature and ventilation
- Medications of patients and their associated effects

Assessment and Outcome Measures
It is essential to;

- set and evaluate the effectiveness of an exercise programme
- provide objective feedback to the patient
- facilitate evidence based practice

Measures can be used as both a baseline measure and exit outcome measure. These may include;

- HR and BP @ rest and during exercise

- RPE
- Body weight
- BMI
- Waist circumference

Measures of functional capacity;

- 6MWT
- Shuttle walk test
- Chester step test

4. PHYSIOTHERAPY IN GERIATRIC CONDITIONS

Rehabilitation is an essential component of geriatric care and therapy and it can make a critical difference in the life quality of elderly people. The recovery of younger adults is different from the geriatric rehabilitation and has some particularities. It is a more difficult and slow progressive process and it must be adapted to the physiological age related decline and co-morbidities.

The goal of rehabilitation in older people is the development of physical independence and the ability to do as many as possible daily living activities.

The following aspects must be taken into account in the rehabilitation of geriatric patients:

- Reactivation - immobilized elderly persons must develop their autonomy as much as possible and must acquire the ability to take care of themselves, focusing on restitutio ad optimum and not on restitutio ad integrum as the younger patients.
- Social reintegration – Elderly patients must return to family and friends, avoiding isolation
- Reinstatement into society, participating to moderate professional activities, other low physical demand activities (walking, hand crafts) or hobbies (e.g. gardening) corresponding to their residual capacity.

The geriatric rehabilitation program starts with episodes of acute care, followed by the transfer of the patient in rehabilitation services and ends with release from all care. Without continued physical activity, the patient is at risk for decline, deconditioning, disuse and use of acute care again.

Curative recovery in the elderly can be rarely achieved in order to allow the return to the usual life style. In patients with chronic diseases or stabilized disabilities the aim is to improve or to prevent further degradation by conservative recovery. In patients with self-service capability jeopardized, preventive recovery can stop the deteriorative process.

The general indications of geriatric rehabilitation are:

- Acute reversible or partially reversible insults e.g. amputation
- Chronic progressive disabling diseases e.g. ostheoarthritis, Parkinson disease
- Acute disabling event due to a chronic disease e.g. stroke due to cerebrovascular disease or hip fracture due to osteoporosis.

Patients unlikely to benefit from rehabilitation are:

- The terminal care patients
- Medically unstable patients, requiring frequent medical review, investigations or changing treatments
- Irrecoverable mental changes, rehabilitation being cooperation and learning process
- Acute febrile illnesses or exacerbation of chronic diseases
- Neoplasias
- Cachectic states,
- Pacemaker wearers
- Hemorrhagic states
- Chronic diseases at the limit of organ failure

A basic principle of geriatric rehabilitation is the individualization of the treatment with adaptation of the physiotherapy programs for each patient regarding the following aspects:

- Age-related functional deficiencies
- Coexisting diseases and the associated treatment
- Remaining capacity, reserves and ability to adapt to exercise
- Previous physical training
- Everyday gestures that the patient can do by himself

- Psychological and intellectual capabilities

- Profession and Hobbies
- Living conditions and social factors
- Financial possibilities

Therapeutic exercises to be done:
Broadly conceived, are designed to improve physical functioning of the geriatric patients and to optimize strength, balance and endurance. The exercise program respects the principle: maximum effect - minimal risk, given the diminished cardiac reserve and risk of hypertension, tachycardia, and coronary ischemic accidents. The program will include muscle exercises compatible with a charge of 75% from the capacity of the cardiovascular system, following the rule "little and often" using sequences of harmonious, rhythmic and comprehensible movements, close to the natural movements of the elderly people.

The following exercises are prohibited in geriatric patients:

- Exercises requiring maximal and submaximal muscular efforts,
- Isometric exercises,
- Extended efforts with the glottis closed,
- Anaerobic exercises,
- Exercises with heavy weights,
- Exercises with the head down below the trunk,
- Exercises with sudden changes of position.

The goal of the geriatric rehabilitation is the recovery and the development of personal independence and the ability to do as many as possible daily living activities. Special programs must be designed for the older people involving an interdisciplinary approach because geriatric rehabilitation must be adapted to

1) The physiological age related decline including sensory impairments, mental status deficiency, depression or dementia, physical inactivity, lack of endurance, impaired balance

2) Multiple coexisting chronic diseases

3) Constrained finances,

4) Lack of social and sometimes family support.

The program must be targeted to the patient's needs and guided by the individual's goals and implies gradual physical activity along with psychological and social recovery.

5. PHYSIOTHERAPY IN OBSTETRICS & GYNAECOLOGICAL CONDITIONS

Obstetrics concerns itself with pregnancy, labour, delivary and the care of the mother after child birth.

*Gynaecology*is the study of disease associated with women which in effect means condition involving the female genital tract.

Physiotherapy in obstetrics condition

From the moment of conception pregnancy profoundly alters the women physiology. There is change in all body system to fulfill the requirement of the body.

Therapeutic exercises may be prescribed to pregnant women for several reasons:

- Primary conditioning unrelated to pregnancy.
- Impairments related to physiological changes of pregnancy, such as back pain, faulty posture, or leg cramps.
- Physical & physiological benefits.
- Preventive measures

Types of exercise

1. Prenatal exercises
2. Preparation for labor
3. Postnatal exercises

Goals:

- Improve posture & correct body mechanics
- Train & strengthen postural muscle
- Teach correct body mechanics in all position
- Prepare for circulatory compromise
- Improve awareness & control of pelvic floor musculature
- Maintain abdominal muscle function & correct diastesis recti
- Provide information about pregnancy & associated problem
- Improve relaxation skill

General Guidelines for Exercise Instruction

- Exercise regularly, at least thrice a week
- Avoid ballistic movements & rapid change in directions.
- Include warm-up & cool down session
- Avoid an anaerobic pace.
- Strenuous activities should be avoided.
- Avoid prolong period of standing especially in third trimester.
- Adequate caloric intake, increase to 300 kcal./day for ex. during pregnancy & 500 kcal./day for exercise during lactation.
- Low resistance & high repetitions ex. is recommended, avoid Valsalva maneuvers.
- Stop exercise if any unusual symptoms occur.

Absolute contraindications

- Pregnancy Induced HTN BP >140/90 mmHg.
- Diagnosed heart disease IHD, RHD, CHF.
- Premature rupture of membrane.
- Placental abruption.
- History of preterm delivery.
- Recurrent miscarriage.
- Persistent vaginal bleeding.
- Fetal distress.
- Incomplete cervix
- Thrombophlebitis & pulmonary embolism.
- Pre-eclampsia
- polyhydraminos / oligohydraminos
- Acute infection

Relative contraindications

- Diabetes
- Anemia's or other blood disorders
- Thyroid disorder
- Dilated cervix
- Extreme obesity / underweight
- Breech presentation during third trimester
- Multiple gestation
- Exercise induced asthma

- Peripheral vascular disease
- Pain of any kind

Physiotherapy in gynaecological conditions:
Infections such as: vulvitis, vaginitis, cervicitis, salphingitis, PID (Pelvic Inflammatory Diseases).
Treatment: In acute phase - chemotherapy; in chronic phase- pulsed or continuous SWD

Cyst & new growth: treated with pulsed SWD /US for softning of painful abdominal muscles adhesion.

Stress incontinence: treated with pelvic floor exercises.

Genital prolapse such as: cystocele, urethrocele, rectocele, enterocele, uterine prolapsed. Treatment: pelvic floor strengthing exercises

Menstrual disorder: treated with pain coping strategies, relaxation & breathing techniques and TENS.

Backache & abdominal pain: treated with TENS.

6. *PHYSIOTHERAPY IN SPORTS & FITNESS*

The team physiotherapist has become one of the most important assets any coach can have when working with a team. The physiotherapist brings dynamics to the warming up, conditioning, muscle activation as well as the recovery of the players. Due to the high intensity of matches, tournaments and training sessions a scientific approach towards the correct prevention, management and rehabilitation of sport injuries has became a necessity when managing any team.

Definition of the Sports Physiotherapist in team sport:
The basic function of a Physiotherapist in Sport is the application of treatment by physical means: electrical, thermal, mechanical, hydraulic, and manual therapeutic exercises with special techniques. The Physiotherapist in Sport focuses its objectives in the field of sport and physical activity.

Based on the definition of the WCPT * on Physiotherapy in Sport, this is the set of methods, techniques and performances, which through the use and application of physical agents prevent, recover and readjust a person with sport or exercise injuries at different levels.

Role of the team Physiotherapist
- Assessment and Treatment of acute and chronic injuries on rest days.
- Stretching before training or matches.

- Muscle activation before training and matches.
- Pre match strapping / treatments.
- Medical cover at training sessions and matches.
- Medical screening and injury prevention.
- Liaising with management regarding the severity of injuries and the conditioning of the team.
- Referral for Scans / Surgery.
- Rehabilitation of the injured player.
- Recovery sport massages, hydrotherapy pool sessions and recovery ice-baths or contrast baths after matches.
- Psychological support during tournaments and matches.

1. **Assessment and treatment of acute and chronic injuries:**

    - *Acute Injuries require early assessment and intervention*
    – Anti inflammatory treatment modalities.
    – Importance of compression and ice
    – Intensive Physiotherapy, strengthening, mobility and regaining function.
    – Rehabilitation of the injury and maintenance of full body strength.
    – Prevention of recurrence by giving home exercises, stretching and proprioception exercises
    - *Chronic Injuries*
    – Ongoing management and training modifications
    – Ongoing rehabilitation

2. **Stretching and muscle activation before training or matches:**

    - The physiotherapist is a specialist in the field of applying the correct stretching and stretching methods to prevent injury during the team warm up prior to a game.
    - The use of evidence based muscle activation techniques to activate local and global muscle stabilisers before a game.

3. **Pre-Match Strapping and Treatment:**

    - A large percentage of players use prophylactic strapping.
    - The application of kinematic taping for muscle activation.

• Numerous players are playing with injuries and require treatment pre-match to improve performance.

4. **Medical Cover at Matches and Training:**

   • Immediate Medical Management on the Field of play.
   • Assessment and decision making on continuing play.
   • Management of blood injuries, sprains, contusions and hydration of the players.

5. **Medical Screening and Injury Prevention:**

   • Based on previous injuries and medical history of the player.
   • Biomechanical assessment identifying weak links and treatment / rehabilitation programme.
   • In season prehabilitation sessions twice a week, small groups on rotation.
   • Individual sessions.

6. **Liaising with Management and Conditioning of the team:**

   • Introducing players back from injury.
   • Reducing volume for players with chronic injuries
   • Building preventative exercises into gym routines.
   • Fitness to play
   • Medical responsibility to the player.

7. **Referral for Scans and Surgery:**

   • Close links with hospitals and consultants.
   • Using only the best surgeons in the region.
   • Able to refer at short notice.
   • Discussions and joint management of athlete to ensure a quick and safe return to training / playing.

8. **Rehabilitation:**

The Physiotherapist's aim, after recovering from injury, is to put all his effort into the regaining of muscle strength and mobility. The Physiotherapist in Sport should regain the functionality of the athlete as quickly as possible, accelerating the biological processes of recovery from injury, limiting his training as little as possible and ensure that they are reinstated into the team, with the greatest prospects for success

9. **Recovery after matches:**

   - Cool down and after match stretching.
   - Sport massages.
   - Hydrotherapy pool sessions.
   - Recovery ice-baths or contrast baths after matches.

10. **Psychological Support:**

    - The player feels isolated when he is injured.
    - Players spend a great deal of time in Rehab Centre.
    - Long term injured players spend more time with medics than team mates.
    - Injured players will talk to medics about things they will not mention to other members of the management team.
    - Players know that conversations with the medical staff are confidential.

CHAPTER FOUR

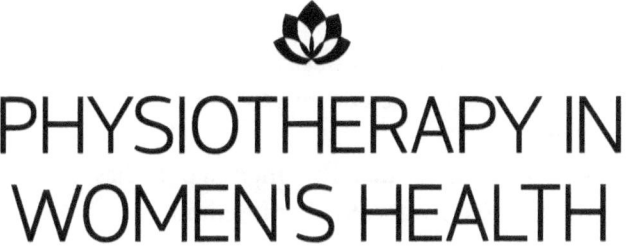

PHYSIOTHERAPY IN WOMEN'S HEALTH

1. *ANATOMY OF FEMALE REPRODUCTIVE TRACT*

The internal organs of the female reproductive system lie in the pelvic cavity and consist of the vagina, uterus, uterine tubes and two ovaries.

v. **Vagina**

The vagina is an elastic, muscular tube that connects the cervix of the uterus to the exterior of the body. It is located inferior to the uterus and posterior to the urinary bladder.
The vagina has three layers: - an outer covering of areolar tissue, a middle layer of smooth muscles and inner lining of stratified squamous epithelium that forms ridges.

- **Functions of the vagina :-**

The vagina functions as the receptacle for the penis during sexual intercourse and carries sperm to the uterus and fallopian tubes. It also serves as the birth canal by stretching to allow delivery of the foetus during childbirth. During menstruation, the menstrual flow exits the body via the vagina.

v. **Ovaries**

The <u>ovaries</u> are a pair of small glands about the size and shape of almonds, located on the left and right sides of the pelvic body cavity lateral to the superior portion of the uterus. They are 2.5 to 3.5 cm long, 2 cm wide and 1cm thick.

The ovaries have two layers of tissue:-

The medulla: - this liesin the centre and consists of fibrous tissue, blood **vessels** and nerves.

The cortex: - this surrounds the medulla. It has a frame work of connective tissue covered by germinal epithelium.

- **Function of ovaries:** - Ovaries produce female sex hormones such as estrogen and progesterone as well as ova (commonly called "eggs"), the female gametes. Ova are produced from oocyte cells that slowly develop throughout a woman's early life and reach maturity after puberty. Each month during ovulation, a mature ovum is released. The ovum travels from the ovary to the fallopian tube, where it may be fertilized before reaching the uterus.

v. *Fallopian Tubes (uterine tubes)*

The <u>fallopian tubes</u> are a pair of muscular tubes that extend from the left and right superior corners of the uterus to the edge of the ovaries. It has about 10cm long. They lie in the upper free border of the broad ligament and their trumpet – shaped lateral ends penetrate the posterior wall, opening into the peritoneal cavity close to the ovaries. The end of each tube has small finger-like projections called fimbriae. The <u>fimbriae</u> swipe over the outside of the ovaries to pick up released ova and carry them into the infundibulum for transport to the uterus. The inside of each fallopian tube is covered in cilia that work with the smooth muscle of the tube to carry the ovum to the uterus. Fertilization of the ovum usually takes place in the uterine tube.

v. *Uterus*

The <u>uterus</u> is a hollow, muscular, pear-shaped organ located posterior and superior to the urinary bladder. Connected to the two fallopian tubes on its superior end and to the vagina (via the <u>cervix</u>) on its inferior end, the uterus is also known as the womb, as it surrounds and supports the developing foetus during pregnancy. The inner lining of the uterus, known as the <u>endometrium</u>, provides support to the embryo during early development.

The parts of the uterus are the fundus, body and cervix. Vagina is the openings of the uterine tubes.

The fundus: - this is the dome shaped part of the uterus above the openings of the uterine tubes.

The body: - this is the main part. It is narrowest inferiorly at the interna os where it is continuous with the cervix.

The cervix:- (neck of the uterus) this protrudes through the anterior wall of the vagina, opening into it at the external os.

It has composed of three layers:-

Perimetrium: - this is peritoneum, which is disrtributed differently on the various surfaces of the uterus.

Myometrium :- this is the thickest layer of tissue in the uterine wall.it is a mass of smooth muscle fibres interlaced with areolar tissue, blood vessels and nerves

Endometrium :- this consist of columnar epithelium containing a large number of mucus secreting tubular glands.

The visceral muscles of the uterus contract during childbirth to push the fetus through the birth canal.

v. *Vulva*

The <u>vulva</u> is the collective name for the external female genitalia located in the pubic region of the body. The vulva surrounds the external ends of the urethral opening and the vagina and includes the mons pubis, labia majora, labia minora, and clitoris.

The mons pubis, or pubic mound, is a raised layer of adipose tissue between the skin and the <u>pubic bone</u> that provides cushioning to the vulva. The inferior portion of the mons pubis splits into left and right halves called the <u>labia majora</u>. The mons pubis and labia majora are covered with pubic hairs. Inside of the labia majora are smaller, hairless folds of skin called the <u>labia minora</u> that surround the vaginal and urethral openings. On the superior end of the labia minora is a small mass of erectile tissue known as the clitoris that contains many nerve endings for sensing sexual pleasure.

v. *Breasts and Mammary Glands*

The **breasts** are specialized organs of the female body that contain mammary glands, milk ducts, and adipose tissue. The two breasts are located on the left and right sides of the thoracic region of the body. In the center of each breast is a highly pigmented **nipple** that releases milk when stimulated. The areola, a thickened, highly pigmented band of skin that surrounds the nipple, protects the underlying tissues during breastfeeding. The **mammary glands** are a special type of sudoriferous glands that have been modified to produce milk to feed infants. Within each breast, 15 to 20 clusters of mammary glands become active during pregnancy and remain active until milk is no longer needed. The milk passes through milk ducts on its way to the nipple, where it exits the body. Lactation is stimulated by the harmone prolactin.

2. GENDER DIFFERENCES IN MUSCLE MORPHOLOGY

- There are number of ways to compare the gender difference in strength & even greater number of why these differences exist.
  - There are several obvious differences between men and women, including the following:

1. An average man is **taller 3-4 inches than** an average woman.
2. Men have **more bodily hair** than women do, especially on the chest and extremities
3. Men are over **30% stronger than women**, especially in the upper body. Although many feminists cannot face this fact, females simply do not have the strength or endurance necessary to be, for example, effective combat soldiers.
4. On average, girls begin **puberty changing approximately two years before** boys.
5. Men have **larger hearts and lungs,** and **their higher levels of testosterone** cause them to produce greater amounts of red blood cells.
6. Differences in intake and delivery of oxygen translate into some aspects of performance: when a man is jogging at about 50% of his capacity, a woman will need to work at over 70% of her capacity to keep up with him.
7. Female fertility decreases after age 35, ending with menopause, but men are capable of making children even when very old.

8. Men's skin has more collagen and sebum, which makes it thicker and oiler than women's skin.
9. Women generally have a greater body fat percentage than men.
10. Men and women have different levels of certain hormones; for example, men have a higher concentration of androgens such as testosterone, while women have a higher concentration of estrogens.
11. An average male brain has approximately 4% more cells and 100 grams more brain tissue than an average female brain. This is not connected with intelligence! Research points to no overall difference in intelligence between males and females. However, both sexes have similar brain weight to body weight ratios.
12. In men, the second digit is often shorter than the fourth digit, while in females the second tends to be longer than the fourth.
13. Men have better distance vision and depth perception, and usually better vision in lighted environments. Women have better night vision, see better at the red end of the light spectrum, and have better visual memory

Males

- The skull size is larger.
- The bony mass or the thickness of the bone: thicker.
- Forehead: In males the forehead is slightly sloping or receding.
- Vault of the skull:
- Males: The vault of the skull is more rounded.
- Supraorbital margin:
- Males: More rounded.
- Tympanic plate:
- Males: Larger and the margins are rounded.
- Frontal bone and Forehead:
- Males: Brow Ridges are well demarcated
- Contour of the face:

- Males: The overall length of the skull is longer and the chin is bigger and projects more forwards, the skull is rugged due to its muscular makeup, and the zygomatic bones are also more massive.
- Mastoid Process:
- Males: Large Mastoid process

Females

- The skull size is smaller comparatively.

The bony mass or the thickness of the bone: thinner.

- Females: The forehead is vertical.
- Females: The vault is flattened than that in females.
- Females: Sharp.
- Females: Smaller and the margins are less rounded.
- Females: Smooth more vertical Frontal bone
- Females: The skull is rounded, with the facial bones being smoother, with both the jaws mandible and the maxilla being smaller.
- Females: Small Mastoid process

SKELETAL DIFFERENCES
PELVIS:

- Broader flatter in females
- Rounder pelvic inlet
- Whereas in male pelvis is narrow and 'v' shape pelvic inlet.

PHYSIOLOGICAL CHANGES
MALE

- Male sex hormones:

- Androgens
- Testosterone.

- These hormones are important for muscle fibre and strength development.
- They are anabolic and contribute to muscle hypertrophy and decreasing body fat percentage.
- Muscle> fat

FEMALE
Female sex hormones:

- estrogens
- Estradiol
- Progesteron.
- estrogen a hormone that can interfere with potentials for muscle growth by increasing body fat stores. These factors together help us understand why women do not make muscle size gains that are comparable to those of men.
- Fat> muscle

STRENGTH
IN MALES:

- Men appear to demonstrate larger absolute increases in strength and degree of muscle hypertrophy than women when both undergo identical weight training regimens.
- Men showed greater relative strength increase than women because muscle cross-sectional area is directly related to ability to produce force.

IN FEMALES:

- Women have lower proportion of their total lean body mass in their upper body so this may warrant additional upper strength training.
- An average woman responds to weight training with slight increase in muscle girth and decrease in intramuscular and subcutaneous fat stores, little change in limb circumference.
- Muscle cross sectional area is two times greater in males than females in body builders.

Women gain relative strength at the same rate as men when performing identical resistance training programme because women begins weight training regimes at lower resistances than men.
Women are more flexible than men.

- Depending on the type of pelvis they inherit, women with broader and shallower pelvis have greater range of motion in hips.
- Women also have greater elbow extension because of shorter upper arc in olecranon process than men.

3. ANEMIA IN PREGNANCY

Anemia is the commonest, haematological disorder that may occur in pregnancy. It is a reduction in the oxygen carrying capacity of the blood, which may be due to:

- A reduced number of red blood cells
- A low concentration of hemoglobin, or
- A combination of both.

Classification of anemia

v. Physiological anemia
v. Pathological anemia

- Iron deficiency
- Folic acid deficiency
- Vitamin B12 deficiency
- Protein deficiency

v. Hemorrhagic anemia

- Acute- following bleeding in early months of pregnancy or APH
- Chronic- hookworm infestation, bleeding piles, etc.

v. Hemolytic anemia

- Familial- congenital acholuric jaundice, sickle cell anemia, etc.
- Acquired- malaria, severe infection, etc.
- Bone marrow insufficiency- hypoplasia or aplasia due to radiation, drugs or severe infection.
- Hemoglobinopathies.

Iron deficiency anemia

About 95% of pregnant women with anemia have the iron deficiency type. A pregnant woman is said to be anemic if her haemoglobin is less than 10gm percent.

Causes

- Reduced intake or absorption of iron- this includes dietary deficiency and gastrointestinal disturbances such as morning sickness.
- Excess demand such as multiple pregnancies, chronic inflammation particularly of the urinary tract.
- Decreased absorption due to decreased gastric acidity and dietary imbalance

Signs and symptoms

- Pallor of mucous membranes
- Lassitude and feeling of weakness
- Giddiness
- Tachycardia and palpitations
- Dyspnea
- Anorexia and indigestion
- Swelling of the legs

Effects of anemia on the mother

- Reduced resistance to infection caused by impaired cell-mediated immunity.
- Reduced ability to withstand postpartum hemorrhage

Effects of anemia on the fetus

- Increased risk of intrauterine hypoxia and growth retardation
- Pre-maturity
- Low birth-weight
- Anemia a few months later birth due to poor stores
- Increased risk of perinatal morbidity and mortality

Management

In the tropics, majority of cases with anemia in pregnancy have a low socioeconomic status.

Prophylaxis

- Avoidance of frequent childbirths- a minimum interval between pregnancies, should be at least two years, to replenish the iron lost

during childbirth and lactation
- Supplementary iron therapy- daily administration of 200mg of ferrous sulphate along with 1mg of folic acid is quite effective prophylactic procedure.
- Dietary advice- a balanced diet, rich in iron and protein, which is affordable by the woman and easily digestible, should be recommended.
- Adequate treatments to eradicate illness likely to cause anemia- these are hook worm infestation, dysentery, bleeding piles, and malaria and urinary tract infections.
- Early detection of falling hemoglobin level- hemoglobin level should be estimated at the first antenatal visit, at 28th and finally 36th week.

Curative management

Women having haemoglobin level of 7.5 mg percent and those with associated obstetrical- medical complications even with moderate degree of anaemia should be hospitalized. Following therapeutic measures are to be instituted.

- Diet – a balanced diet, which is rich in protein, iron and vitamins.
- Appropriate antibiotic therapy to eradicate even a minimal septic focus
- Effective therapy to cure the disease contributing to the cause of anemia
- Iron therapy to raise the hemoglobin level and to restore the iron reverse at least in part, if possible, before the woman goes into labor

This may be oral iron or parenteral iron depending on the severity of anemia, duration of pregnancy and associated complicating factors.

4. *ANTENATAL CARE*

Antenatal care Systematic supervision [examination and advice] of a woman during pregnancy is called antenatal/prenatal care. It comprises of:

- Careful history taking and examination [general and obstetrical].
- Advice given to pregnant woman.

Procedure at the subsequent visits
Generally check up is done at the interval of 4 weeks up to 28 weeks; at interval of 2 weeks upto36 weeks and thereafter weekly till delivery.

WHO recommended, visit may be curtailed to at least 4; first in second trimester around 16 weeks, second between 24-28 weeks, third visit at 32 weeks and the fourth visit at 36 weeks.

Examination of Maternal health

General:- In each visit weight, pallor, odema legs and blood pressure are checked and recorded.

Abdominal examination:

Inspection:- Abdominal enlargement, pregnanacy marks-linea nigra, striae, surgical scars [midline or suprapubic]

Palpation:- To note the height of the fundus above the symphsis pubis.

Vaginal examination:- Vaginal examination is done in the later months of pregnancy [beyond 37 weeks].

Fetal Health

To check fetal growth, fundal height, fetal heart rate, amniotic fluid volume, presentation and fetal activity.

Antenatal advice

Principles:-

- To counsel the woman about the importance of regular check up.
- To maintain or improve, the health status of the woman and advice her regarding diet, drugs, and hygiene.
- To improve the psychology and to remove the fear of unknown by counseling the woman.

Diet:-

The diet during pregnancy should be adequate to provide:

- Good maternal health.
- Optimum fetal growth.
- To strengthen vitality required during pregnancy.
- Successful lactation.

The increased calorie requirement is to the extent of 300 over the non-pregnancy state during the second half of pregnancy. Woman with normal BMI should eat adequately so as to gain the optimum weight {11kg}. The pregnancy diet ideally should be light, nutritious, easily digestible, and rich in proteins, minerals and vitamins.

Supplementary nutritional therapy:-

Supplementary iron therapy is needed for all pregnant mothers from 16 weeks onwards. Above 10gm% of hb,1 tab of ferrous sulphate {fersolate} containing 60 mg of iron is enough. The dose should be proportionately increased with lower haemoglobin level to 2-3 tab {45mg} a day. Suplementary vitamins are given daily from 20th week onwards.

Antenatal hygiene

- **Rest and sleep:-** Excessive and strenuous work should be avoided specially in first trimester and last 4 weeks. The client should be in bed for about 10 hrs{8hrs at night and 2hrs at noon}specially in last 6 weeks. In late pregnancy lateral posture is more comfortable.
- **Bowel:-** Constipation is common. Regular bowel movement may be facilitated by regulation of diet taking plenty of fluids, vegetables, milk or prescribed stool softeners at bed time.
- **Bathing:-** The client should take daily bath but be careful regarding slipping in the bathroom due to imbalance.
- **Clothing,shoes and belt:-** The client should wear loose but comfortable garments. High heels should be avoided. Constricting belt should also be avoided.
- **Care of breasts:-** Breast engorgement can cause discomfort during late pregnancy. A well fitting brassiere can give relief.
- **Coitus:-** women with increased risk of miscarriage or preterm labour should avoid coitus. Generally coitus is not restricted during pregnancy.
- **Smoking and alchol:-** Smoking and alcohol consumption should be avoided during pregnancy as its injurious to mother as well as fetal health. It may lead to abortion, maldevelopment or growth restriction.
- **Travel:-** Travel by vehicles having heavy jerks are to be avoided specially in first trimester and the last 6 weeks. Travel in aircraft is safe upto 36 weeks. Air travel is contraindicated in case of placenta praevia, pre-eclampsia, severe anaemia and sickle cell disease.

Immunization:-

Tetnus: 0.5 ml tetnus toxoid is given intramuscularly at 6 weeks interval of 2 such, the first one is to be given between 16 -24 weeks. Women who are immunized in the past, a booster dose of 0.5 ml is given in the last trimester.

GENERAL ADVICE:

- The patient should be persuaded to attend the antenatal check up positively on the scheduled date of visit.
- She is instructed to report to the physcisn if any untoward symptoms arise like intense headache, disturbed sleep with restlessness, urinary troubles, epigastric pain, vomiting and scanty urine.

She is advised to come to the hospital in following circumstances:-

1. Painful uterine contraction at interval of about 10 minutes or earlier and continued for at least 1 hour -suggestive onset of labour.
2. Sudden gush of watery fluid per vaginum - suggestive of premature rupture of membranes.
3. Active vaginal bleeding.

5. HYPERTENSION IN PREGNANCY

Hypertension is one of the common disorders of pregnancy and contributes to the maternal and perinatal morbidity and mortality.

Classification of hypertension in pregnancy

A . Pregnancy induced hypertension

1. With proteinurea and/or edema

- Preeclampsia
- Eclampsia

2. Without gross edema or proteinurea

- Gestational hypertension.

B . Chronic hypertension in pregnancy
Preganancy is unrelated to the hypertensive state

1. Essential hypertension.
2. Renovascular hypertension
3. Pheochromocytoma
4. Coarctation of aorta
5. Connective tissue disease-systemic lupus erythematosus.

C. Hypertension worsened by pregnancy

1. Superimposed preeclampsia
2. Superimposed eclampsia.

Pregnancy induced hypertension

The hypertension develops as a direct result of the gravid state. The clinical types of PIH are:

- *Preeclampsia*
- *Eclampsia*
- *Gestational hypertension*

Preeclampsia:

Preeclampsia is characterized by development of hypertension to the extent of 140/90 mm Hg with proteinurea induced by pregnancy after the 20th week in a previously normotensive and non-proteinuric woman.

Classifaction of preeclampsia

Mild preeclampsia: Blood pressure- more than 140/90 mm Hg but less than 160/110 mm Hg without proteinurea.

Svere preeclampsia: blood pressure exceeds 160/100mm Hg with an increase in proteinurea (75gm per day) and where edema is marked.

Symptoms and signs:

- Frontal headache
- Disturbed sleep
- Diminished urinary output
- Epigastric pain associated with vomiting
- Blurring or dumness of vision or at times complete blindness (vision is usually regained 4-6 hrs following delivery)
- A rapid gain in weight of more than 2.5kg a month
- Scanty liquor or growth retardation of the fetus.

Complications
During pregnancy:

- Eclampsia 2 percent
- Placental abruption and intrauterine fetal death

- Oliguria and anuria
- Dimness of vision and blindness
- Preterm labor
- HELLP Syndrome

During labor:

- Eclampsia
- Postpartum hemorrhage

Puerperium

- Eclampsia
- Shock (related to reduced sodium and chloride)
- Sepsis

Management
Rest : the woman should be in bed preferably in left lateral position as much as possible to lesser the effects of venacaval compression. Rest increases the renal blood flow causing increased diuresis, increases the uterine blood flow causing improved placental perfusion and reduces the blood pressure.
Diet : a diet rich in protein, fiber and vitamins is recommended. Omission of extra salty food and extra salt in the dish is desirable. Fish oil in pregnancy may act as an antipalteley agent, thereby preventing hypertension and proteinuric preeclampsia.
Antihypertensive therapy: the commonest oral drugs are
Methyldopa 0.5-2 gm/day
Labetalol 200mh six to eight hourly.
If blood pressure is not under control, nifedipine, a calcium channel blocker 10-20 mg twice a day or hydralazine 25 mg twice are added.
Sedatives: mild sdatives are given to reduce the emotional factor that contributes to elevation of blood pressure. Phenobarbitone 60mg or diazepam 5mg are given.
Laxative: if thewoman is constipated, a mild laxative like milk of magnesia 4 teaspoons may be given.
Obstetric management : in cases with pregnancy beyond 37th completed week or where the condition fails to improve within 6-8 hours , delivery

should be considered irrespective to the period gestation. Termination is done depending on the Bishops score, either by low rupture of the membranes aided by oxytocin infusion or by cesarean section.

HELLP Syndrome: the syndrome of hemolysis elevated liver enzymes and low platelet count is a rare complication of PIH. The syndrome is manifested by nausea, vomiting , epigastric or upper right quadrant pain along with biochemical and hematological changes. Pregnancies complicated by HELLP syndrome have been associated with both poor maternal and poor fetal outcome.

Serious maternal morbidity includes: disseminated intravascular coagulation, acute renal failure, pulmonary edema, subcapsular liver hematomaand retinal detachement.

Diagnosis :

- heamolysis – abnormal blood picture, increased bilirubin, increased lactic dehydrogenase.
- Elevated liver enzymes
- Low platelets.

Treatment : in pregnancies less than 34 weeks gestation, conservative treatment is given using plasma volume expanders and vasodilators. In term pregnancies and where there is a deteriorating maternal or fetal condition, immediate delivery is recommended.

Eclampsia

Preeclampsia when complicated with convulsion and/or coma is called eclampsia .it is more common in primigravidae , five times more common in twins than in singleton pregnancies and occurs between the 36th week and term in more than 50%.

Onset of convulsions

Convulsions occur more frequently beyond 36th week.

- Antepartum (50%) : fits occur before the onset of labor
- Intrapartum (30%) fits occur for the first time during laor.
- Postpartum (20%): fits occur for the first time in puerperium, usually within 48 hrs of delivery.

Eclamptic convulsions

The convulsions are epileptiform and consist of four stages.

Premonitory stage- the patient becomes unconscious. There is twitching of the muscles of the face, tongue and limbs. This stage last for 30 seconds.

Tonic stage- the whole body goes in a tonic stage. Respiration ceases and the tongue protrudes between the teeth. Eyeballs become fixed . this lasts for about 30 seconds.

Clonic stage- all the voluntary muscles undergo alternative contraction and relaxation. This stage lasts for 1-4 minutes.

Stage coma- it may lasts for a brief period or may persist until another convulsion. At times, the patient appears to be in a confused state following the fit and fails to remember the happenings.

<u>*Complications of eclampsia*</u>

Injuries- tongue bite, injuries due to falling out of bed.
Cardiovascular- vasospasm, pulmonary embolism
Renal- oliguria, renal failure
Hematological- hypovolumia, thrombocytopenia
Neurological- cerebral edema , cerebral hemorrhage
Respiratory- pneumonia
Sensory- disturbed vision

Management

The aims of immediate management in the hospital are to:

- Clear and maintain the airway
- Prevent hypoxia
- Prevent injury
- Arrest convulsions
- Effect delivery in 6-8 hours

Anticonvulsant therapy- Magnesium sulphate is the drug of choice.

Antihypertensives and diuretics- Hydralazine 5mg is given inravenously. Labetalol is given by slow IV route 20md per hour.

Gestational hypertension

Gestational hypertension is a sustained rise of blood pressure to 140/90 mmHg or more on two occasions , 4 or more hours apart beyond the 20th week of pregnancy or during the first 24hrs after delivery in a previously normotensive woman.

The hypertension may be a stress response. These patients are more likely to develop hypertension with the use of oral contraceptives or in subsequent pregnancies.

Chronic hypertension in pregnancy

Chronic hypertension disease is defined as the presence of hypertension of any cause before the 20th week of pregnancy.

Chronic hypertension has two causes:

- It may be a long term problem, present before the beginning of pregnancy.
- It may be secondary to existing medical problems such as

1. Renal disease
2. Systemic lupus erythematosus
3. Coarctation of the aorta
4. Cushing's syndrome
5. Pheocromocytoma

The perinatal morbidity and mortality are increased in those women who develop svere chronic hypertension.

Essential hypertension in pregnancy

The commonest hypertensive state in pregnancy. Its incidence varies from 1-3 percent.

Diagnosis:

- Rise of blood pressure to the extent of 140/90 mm Hg or more during preganacy prior to the 20th week.
- Presistance of blood pressure even after 3 months following delivery.
- Common in elderly women.
- Presence of pre-pregnant hypertension and often family history.
- Presence of hypertensive retinppathy.

Management:

In mild cases with blood pressure less than 160/100 mm Hg , adequate rest, low salt diet and a sedative (phenobarbitone 60 mg 1-3 times daily) are given.

In svere cases , the patient should be hospitalized and placed in the treatment protocol as described under preeclampsia. Antihypertensive drugs are given only when blood pressure is raised beyond 160/100 mm Hg because the diminished blood pressure may reduce placental perfusion, which may be determined to the fetus.

The prevalence of hypertension increases with age across all race and sex groups

after the fifth decade of life, the incidence of hypertension increases more rapidly in women; thus, women older than 60 years have higher rates of hypertension compared with men.

Etiology and Pathophysiology of Hypertension in Women

Most secondary hypertension generally occurs with equal frequency in women and men. Exceptions include hypertension caused by renal artery stenosis due to fibromuscular dysplasia, which occurs more commonly in women than men, and secondary hypertension due to the use of oral contraceptives, preeclampsia, and vasculitides.

Although there are exceptions in individual patients, hypertensive women tend to have lower plasma renin activity (PRA) than hypertensive men. PRA, intravascular volume, and BP vary during the menstrual cycle in normotensive women. The increase in intravascular volume during the luteal phase of the menstrual cycle may play a role in hypertension in some women and may account in part for hypertension associated with use of oral contraceptives. Karpanou and colleagues demonstrated that premenopausal hypertensive women have increased testosterone levels during ovulation and increased testosterone and PRA during the luteal phase of the menstrual cycle. In this study, hypertensive women with high PRA exhibited no change in BP during the cycle (much like normotensive patients), whereas hypertensive women with relatively low PRA had a nighttime increase in BP during ovulation. The authors speculate that BP may be regulated mainly by the renin-angiotensin-aldosterone system in hypertensive persons with high PRA, whereas sex steroids may play a more important role in those with low PRA.

In premenopausal women, hypertension is often characterized by a higher resting heart rate, left ventricular ejection time, cardiac index, and pulse pressure and a lower total peripheral resistance and total blood volume compared with age-matched men with the same BP level. Hypertension in older women tends to be characterized by elevated peripheral vascular resistance, low or normal plasma volume, and a tendency toward low PRA.

Oral Contraceptives and BP

Many women taking oral contraceptives experience a small but detectable increase in BP; a small percentage experiences the onset of frank hypertension. This is true even with modern preparations that contain only 30 µg estrogen. The Nurses' health study found that person's currently using oral contraceptives had a significantly increased risk of hypertension compared with those who had never used oral contraceptives (relative risk, 1.8; 95% confidence interval, 1.5–2.3). Absolute risk was small: only 41.5 cases of hypertension per 10,000 person years could be attributed to oral contraceptive use. Controlled prospective studies have demonstrated a return of BP to pretreatment levels within 3 months of discontinuing oral contraceptives, indicating that their BP effect is readily reversible.

Oral contraceptives occasionally may precipitate accelerated or malignant hypertension. Family history of hypertension, including pre-existing pregnancy-induced hypertension, occult renal disease, obesity, middle age (>35 years), and duration of oral contraceptive use increase susceptibility to hypertension. Contraceptive-induced hypertension appears to be related to the progestogenic, not the estrogenic, potency of the preparation.

Regular monitoring of BP throughout contraceptive therapy is recommended, and it has been suggested that the duration of prescription contraceptive use be limited to 6 months to ensure at least semiannual reevaluations. Withdrawal of the offending contraceptive agent is generally desirable in cases of contraceptive-induced hypertension, but such therapy may have to be continued in some women (eg, if other contraceptive methods are not suitable) and combined with antihypertensive therapy.

Menopause and BP

The effect of menopause on BP is controversial. Longitudinal studies have not documented a rise in BP with menopause, while cross-sectional studies have found significantly higher SBP and DBP in postmenopausal vs premenopausal women. In NHANES III, the rate of rise in SBP tended to be steeper in postmenopausal compared with premenopausal women until the sixth decade, when the rate of increase tended to slow. Stassen and associates reported that even after adjustment for age and body mass index, postmenopausal women are more than twice as likely to have hypertension as premenopausal women. In a prospective study of conventional and ambulatory BP levels, postmenopausal women had higher SBP (4–5 mm Hg) than premenopausal and perimenopausal controls. the increase in SBP per decade was 5 mm hg greater in the perimenopausal and postmenopausal women than in the premenopausal group. Thus, there is evidence that at least part of the rise in BP (particularly SBP) seen later in life in women is due to menopause. A menopause-related increase in BP has been attributed to a variety of factors, including estrogen withdrawal, overproduction of pituitary hormones, weight gain, or a combination of these and other yet-undefined neurohumoral influences.

Choice of Antihypertensive Drugs for Women

While women generally respond to antihypertensive drugs similarly to men, some special considerations may dictate treatment choices for women. Angiotensin-converting enzyme inhibitors (ACEIs) and angiotensin receptor blockers (ARBs) are contraindicated for women who are or intend to become pregnant because of the risk of fetal developmental abnormalities. Diuretics are particularly useful in elderly individuals because of a decreased risk of hip fracture. some antihypertensive drugs have sex-specific adverse effect profiles. For example, in the Treatment of Mild Hypertension Study (TOMHS), women reported twice as many adverse effects as men. Women are more likely to develop diuretic-induced hyponatremia, and men are more likely to develop gout. Hypokalemia is more common in women taking a diuretic. ACEI-induced cough is twice as common in women as in men, and women are more likely to complain of calcium channel blocker–related peripheral edema and minoxidil-induced hirsutism.

Nonpharmacologic Treatment of Hypertension

Adoption of healthy lifestyles by all persons is critical for the prevention of high BP and is an indispensable part of the management of those with hypertension. Weight loss of as little as 10 lb (4.5 kg) reduces BP and/or prevents hypertension in a large proportion of overweight persons, although maintenance of normal body weight is ideal. BP is also benefited by adoption of the Dietary Approaches to Stop Hypertension (DASH) eating plan, which is a diet rich in fruits, vegetables, and low-fat dairy products with a reduced content of dietary cholesterol as well as saturated and total fat (modification of whole diet). It is rich in potassium and calcium. Dietary sodium should be reduced to no more than 100 mmol/d (2.4 g of sodium). Additional measures include regular aerobic physical activity such as brisk walking at least 45 minutes per day most days of the week. Alcohol intake should be limited to no more than 1 drink per day in women. A drink is 12 oz of beer, 5 oz of wine, or 1.5 oz of 80-proof liquor. For overall cardiovascular risk reduction, patients should be strongly counselled to quit smoking.

6. OSTEOPENIA

Osteo means bone and penia indicates a state of being low in quantity

Definition –Osteopenia refers to bone density that is lower than normal peak density but not low enough to be classified as osteoporosis.

Bone density is a measurement of how dense and strong the bones are. If bone density is low compared to normal peak density, said to have osteopenia.If bone density measurement indicate that bone density is between 1.0 and 2.49s.d below would be expected in the average young man or woman, then is said to have a bone density in osteopenic range.

Having osteopenia means there is a greater risk that as time passes you may develop bone density that is very low compared to normal known as osteoporosis.

Causes of Osteopenia

Bones naturally become thinner as people grow older because,beginning in middle age,existing bone cells are reabsorbed by the body faster than new bone is made. As this occurs, the bones lose minerals, heaviness (mass),and structure, making them weaker and increasing their risk of breaking. All people begin losing bone mass after they reach peak bone density at about 30 years of age. The thicker your bone are at about 30,the longer it takes to develop osteopenia or oesteoporosis.

Osteopenia may also be the result of a one or more other conditions, disease processes,or treatments. Women are far more likely to develop osteopenia and osteoporosis than men. This is because women have a lower peak bone density and because the loss of bone mass speeds up as hormonal changes that take place at the time of menopause.In both men and women,the following things can contribute to osteopenia:

- Eating disorders or metabolic problems that do not allow the body to take in and use enough vitamins and minerals.
- Chemotherapy or medicines such as steroids used to treat a number of conditions,including asthma.
- Exposure to radiation.

Having family history of osteoporosis being thin,being white or Asian,limited physical activity,smoking,drinking cola drinks and drinking excessive amount of alcohol also increases the risk of osteopenia and osteoporosis.

Symptoms of Osteopenia

Osteopenia has no symptoms. No pain or change is noticed as the bone becomes thinner,although the risk of breaking a bone increases as the bone becomes less dense.

Diagnosis of Osteopenia

BONE DENSITY TEST –the most accurate test of bone density is dual energy x-ray absorptiometry,although there are some other methods.

DEXA is a form of X-ray that can detect as little as 2% of bone loss per year.A standard X-ray is not useful in diagnosing osteopenia,because it is not sensitive enough to detect small amounts of bone loss or minor changes in bone density.

Treatment of Osteopenia

- Osteopenia is treated by taking steps to prevent it from progressing to osteoporosis.
- Lifestyle changes can help reduce the bone loss that leads to osteopenia.
- Calcium is the most critical mineral for bone mass.Sources of calcium are milk,and other dairy products,green vegetables,and calcium enriched products.
- Calcium supplement ,combines with vitamin.D that helps body to absorb calcium and other minerals.It is found in eggs,salmon,swordfish,and some fish oils.
- Exercise is important for having strong bones,because bone forms in response to stress.Weight –bearing exercises such as walking,dancing are all good choices.
- In addition to diet and exercise,quitting smoking and avoiding excessive use of alcohol and cola reduce our risk of bone loss.
- There are medicines for treating bone thinning.but these are used if osteopenia have progressed to more serious condition called osteoporosis.
- Medicines that may include bisphosphonates,raloxifene,and hormone replacement.

Prevention of Osteopenia
AIM IS TO MAXIMIZE BONE DENSITY

To maximize bone density,plenty of calcium and Vit.D through diet and by spending little time In sun,get weight bearing exercise on a regular basis,avoid smoke,cola and alcohol.

Teach children to eat healthy, get regular exercise, avoid smoking and alcohol.

If older than 30, balanced diet and regular exercise will help slow the loss of bone density, delay osteopenia, and delay or prevent osteoporosis.

7. OSTEOPOROSIS

The normal bone structure

- The bones in our skeleton are made of a thick outer shell and a strong inner mesh filled with collagen (protein), calcium salts and other minerals.
- The inside of our bone looks like honeycomb, with blood vessels and bone marrow in the spaces between bone.

Definition of osteoporosis

- A progressive systematic skeletal disease characterized by low bone mass and micro-architectural deterioration of bone tissue, with a consequent increase in bone fragility and susceptibility to fracture
- Osteoporosis literally translates as "porous bones"
- Osteoporosis occurs when the holes between bone become bigger, making it fragile and liable to break easily

Osteoporosis – primary causes

- Following a period of balanced bone resorption and bone formation, the destruction of bone begins to exceed the formation of bone; this imbalance leads to a net loss of bone, and the beginning of osteoporosis.
- The risk of fracture increases from 1.5 to 3-fold for every 10% decrease in bone mass.
- Degree of bone loss is defined by comparison with young adult mean bone density
- **Bone mineral density (BMD),** a measure of bone mass divided by bone area, increases with age until peak bone density is achieved. Bone mineral density is correlated highly with bone strength and is therefore used to quantitatively screen and diagnose patients.
- Normal bone density is within 1 SD of the young adult mean

- Osteopenic bone density is between 1 and 2.5 SD below the young adult mean (**T-score** between 1 and 2.5)
- Osteoporosis – Density of bone mineral:Osteoporotic bone density is > 2.5 SD below the young adult mean (**T-score** greater than 2.5)
- Those who fall at the lower end of the young normal range (a T-score of >1 SD below the mean) have low bone density and are considered to be at increased risk of osteoporosis

Osteoporosis - prevalence

- In the USA, the estimated prevalence of osteopenia is 15 million in women and 3 million in men.
- The estimated prevalence of osteoporosis is 8 million in women and 2 million in men.
- Although, osteoporosis affects >10 million individuals in the United States, only 10 to 20% are diagnosed and treated
- Osteopenia and osteoporosis are major public health problems, resulting in substantial morbidity and estimated health costs of >$14 billion annually.

Manifestations of osteoporosis

- Osteoporosis has been termed a silent disease because, until a fracture occurs, symptoms are absent.
- Chief clinical manifestations are vertebral and hip fractures
- Rate of fracture increases exponentially with increasing magnitude of **T-scores**
- About 300,000 hip fractures occur each year in the United States
- Hip fractures are associated with a high incidence of deep vein thrombosis and pulmonary embolism (20 to 50%) and a mortality rate between 5 and 20% during the few months after surgery.

Pathogenesis

- Diminished bone mass can result from:

  1. failure to reach an optimal peak bone mass in early adulthood
  2. increased bone resorption

3. decreased bone formation after peak bone mass has been achieved

- All three of these factors probably play a role in most elderly persons. Low bone mass, rapid bone loss, and increased fracture risk correlate with high rates of bone turnover (ie, resorption and formation).
- In osteoporosis, the rate of formation is inadequate to offset the rate of resorption and maintain the structural integrity of the skeleton

Aging vs. Osteoporosis

- Bone resorption rates appear to be maintained or even to increase with age
- Bone formation rates tend to decrease.
- Loss of template due to complete resorption of trabecular elements or to endosteal removal of cortical bone produces irreversible bone loss.
- Age-related microdamage and death of osteocytes may also increase skeletal fragility
- HOWEVER, Osteoporosis is NOT an inevitable consequence of aging; many persons maintain good bone mass and structural integrity into their 80s and 90s.

Risk factors
Risk factors that cannot be modified include:

- Caucasian race
- Advanced age
- Female sex
- Premature menopause (<45 years)
- Prolonged time (>1 year) without a menstrual period

Conditions associated with osteoporosis:

- Anorexia nervosa
- Malabsorption syndromes
- Excessive secretion of parathyroid hormone
- Excessive secretion of thyroid hormone
- Post-transplantation
- Chronic renal disease

- Chronic liver disease
- Excessive secretion of cortisol (Cushing's syndrome)
- Radiographic evidence of osteopenia or vertebral deformity
- Previous fracture not caused by a major accident
- Cancer
- Significant loss of height or an abnormal bend in the upper spine (thoracic kyphosis)

Risk factors that have the potential to be modified include:

- Cigarette smoking
- Excessive alcohol intake
- Inactivity
- Low body weight
- Poor general health
- Prolonged immobilization

Risk Factor – Female Gender

The greater frequency of osteoporotic fractures in women has many causes:

- Women have lower peak bone mass - at age 35, men have 30 percent more bone mass than women, and they lose bone more slowly as they age
- Women generally have lighter, thinner bones than men to begin with so loss is more significant– also, the smaller periosteal diameter of bones in women also increases skeletal fragility
- The rapid decline in estrogen at menopause is associated with an increase in bone resorption without a corresponding increase in bone formation. This imbalance leads to an accelerated net loss of bone that results in decreased bone strength and ultimately may lead to fractures and osteoporosis. function at menopause (typically after age 50) precipitates such rapid bone loss such that most women meet the criteria for osteoporosis by age 70.

(For ex. Estrogen inhibits IL-2; IL-2 promotes osteoclast activity and therefore, bone resorption)

- Women may also lose bone during the reproductive years, particularly with prolonged lactation.
- Another reason for female predominance is that women live longer than men.

Race. Caucasian and Asian women have lower bone density than blacks by as much as 5 to 10 percent. Until recently it was thought that Caucasian women were at greatest risk for osteoporosis, but a recent large-scale study has found that Hispanic, Asian, and Native American women are at least as likely to have low bone mass as Caucasians. And one-third of African American women are also at risk.

Build. Having a delicate frame or weaker bones predisposes you to a higher fracture risk. Overall muscle tone also plays a role in the likelihood of sustaining an injury.

Onset of Menopause. Undergoing early menopause, naturally or surgically, increases your risk, because you will have reduced levels of estrogen for a longer period of time than you would with normal menopause. Because of the abrupt cessation of estrogen production that accompanies surgical menopause, women whose ovaries are removed (69 percent in one study) tend to show signs of osteoporosis within 2 years after surgery if no hormone replacement therapy is instituted. When medically possible, doctors recommend keeping your ovaries intact in order to maintain estrogen production, even if a hysterectomy (removal of the uterus) is necessary.

Heredity. Having a mother, grandmother, or sister with a diagnosis of osteoporosis or its symptoms ("dowager's hump" or multiple fractures) increases your risk. Body type, as well as a possible genetic predisposition to osteoporosis, can be passed from one generation to the next.

Classification of Osteoporosis

Primary osteoporosis in the elderly can be classified as type I or II:

- Type I (menopausal) osteoporosis occurs mainly in persons aged 51 to 75, is six times more common in women, and is associated with vertebral and Colles' (distal radius) fractures.
- Type II (senescent) osteoporosis occurs in persons > 60, is two times more common in women, and is associated with vertebral and hip fractures.

- Overlap between types I and II is substantial, so this classification is of limited clinical use.

Primary osteoporosis is thought to result from the hormonal changes that occur with age, particularly decreasing levels of sex hormones (estrogen in women, testosterone in men). Several other risk factors are usually contributory.

Secondary osteoporosis may be due to many causes.

Distinguishing secondary osteoporosis is important in patients of all ages, because many of the causes are treatable or have an important effect on prognosis

Manifestations of osteoporosis

1. Vertebral Fractures

- A loss of height may indicate a vertebral compression fracture, which occurs in many patients without trauma or other acute precipitant.
- A persistent low backache, or sudden localized pain, could be a warning sign of compression fractures in the vertebrae of the spine.
- But for many, these breaks cause little pain, and may go undetected for years. For some, the only tip-off is a noticeable loss of height, which can reach as much as 8 inches.
- 2. Osteoporosis – Dorsal kyphosis
- Dorsal kyphosis with exaggerated lordosis (dowager's hump) may result from multiple compression fractures. The hump caused by spine fractures is disfiguring. This is the feature of osteoporosis that is the worst thing for most patients. In severe cases, the ribs can touch the pelvic bones.
- Along with the curve in the spine comes an outward curve of the stomach. Women do not realize that the curvature of the spine means the intestines have nowhere to go except forwards.
- Many women think that they are getting fat, and they go on a diet trying to regain their youthful waistline. If they do successfully lose weight, it will only increase their risk for more osteoporotic fractures.
- Osteoporotic fractures commonly affect the hip because the elderly tend to fall sideways or backwards, landing on this joint. Younger, more agile persons tend to fall forward, landing on the outstretched wrist, thus fracturing the distal radius

Osteoporosis – Diagnosis

Without a fracture or bone density screening there is no way to diagnose the presence of osteoarthritis.

The goal is to get as much information about compounding risk factors:

- A complete history of menstrual function, pregnancy, and lactation should be obtained in women, and a history of sexual function should be obtained in men, in whom decreased libido and erectile dysfunction may be due to low testosterone levels.
- Neurologic deficits and drugs that might increase the risk of falls should be analyzed.
- The family history should include fractures and evidence of endocrinopathy or renal calculi.
- One of the most important predictors of osteoporotic fractures is a history of a fracture after age 40 due to minimal or moderate trauma. In such persons, the fracture risk may be increased several fold.
- The physical examination is often unremarkable. Spinal deformity and tenderness over the lower back should be sought.

X-ray findings are generally insufficient for the screening of primary osteoporosis:

- A normal x-ray of bone cannot reliably measure bone density but is useful to identify spinal factures, explains back pain, height loss or kyphosis.
- X-rays may detect osteopenia only when bone loss is > 30%.
- X-ray findings can also suggest other causes of metabolic bone disease, such as the lytic lesions in multiple myeloma and the pseudofractures characteristic of osteomalacia.

Bone densitometry is the only method for diagnosing or confirming osteoporosis in the absence of a fracture

- The National Osteoporosis Foundation recommends that bone densitometry be performed routinely in all women > 65, particularly in those who have one or more risk factors.
- Densitometry can also be used for monitoring the response to therapy.

Dual energy x-ray absorptiometry (DEXA)

- DEXA measures areal density (ie, g/cm2) rather than true volumetric density.
- The test is non-invasive and involves no special preparation.
- Radiation exposure is minimal, and the procedure is rapid. This is the most popular and accurate test to date and the test only takes about 20 to 40 minutes, with a 5 mrem dose of radiation (a full dental x-ray is 300 mrem).

- Can be used to measure bone mineral density in the spine, hip, wrist, or total body.
- However, the standard apparatus is expensive and not portable. Small DEXA machines that can measure the forearm, finger, or heel are less expensive and are portable.

Screening- Ultrasound Densitometry

Ultrasound densitometry can assess the density and structure of the skeleton and appears to predict fracture risk in the elderly. The apparatus is relatively inexpensive, portable, and uses no radiation but can be used only in peripheral sites (eg, the heel), where bone is relatively superficial. Ultrasound devices measure the speed of sound (SOS), as well as specific changes in sound waves (broadband attenuation or BUA) as they pass through bone. QUS measurements provide information on fracture risk by providing an indication of bone density and possibly also information on the quality of the bone. Ultrasound devices do not expose the patient to ionizing radiation.

Osteoporosis – Treatment & Prevention

- Treatment of the patient with osteoporosis frequently involves management of acute fractures as well as treatment of the underlying disease
- Patients should be thoroughly educated to reduce the likelihood of any risk factors associated with bone loss and falling
- A large body of data indicates that optimal calcium intake reduces bone loss and suppresses bone turnover
- Routine to recommend supplemental vitamin D

- Exercise in young individuals increases the likelihood that they will attain the maximal genetically determined peak bone mass. Meta-analyses of studies performed in postmenopausal women indicate that weight-bearing exercise prevents bone loss but does not appear to result in substantial bone gain
- Osteoporosis does not directly cause death. However, an excess mortality of 10 to 20% occurs in patients with established osteoporosis, particularly those with hip fractures.
- Prevention of osteoporotic fractures is critical to avoid a worldwide, costly epidemic. Prevention programs should be developed for patients at risk and for patients with diagnosed osteoporosis.
- **Antiresorptive therapy:** Persons with low bone mass and multiple risk factors, particularly those who have already had an osteoporotic fracture, should be considered for antiresorptive therapy. Antiresorptive drugs include estrogens, bisphosphonates, selective estrogen receptor modulators, and calcitonin.
- **Estrogen** can prevent menopausal bone loss in most women. Estrogen replacement therapy (ERT) is the treatment of choice for postmenopausal women, particularly those who had an early menopause, and for women who have had a hysterectomy. ERT is particularly effective during the first few years after menopause when bone loss is most rapid. Epidemiologic studies and the few prospective clinical trials of estrogen suggest that ERT or HRT decreases the risk of osteoporotic fractures by 30 to 50%. Because other antiresorptive drugs may have an additive effect when given with estrogen, combination therapy should be considered in patients who have very low bone density, continue to lose bone, or incur a fracture while taking ERT or HRT.
- **Bisphosphonates** are potent antiresorptive drugs that directly inhibit osteoclast activity. For women who cannot tolerate estrogen or have contraindications (eg, preexisting breast cancer, risk factors for breast cancer), bisphosphonates are considered the next choice; these drugs increase bone mass and decrease the risk of fractures, particularly in patients taking glucocorticoids. Bisphosphonates, particularly alendronate, have also decreased the incidence of vertebral and nonvertebral fractures by >= 50% in large cohorts of postmenopausal women.

- Alendronate is used to prevent (5 mg/day) and treat (10 mg/day) osteoporosis. Pamidronate is available IV for treatment of hypercalcemia of malignancy and Paget's disease but has been used in osteoporosis.
- **Selective estrogen receptor modulators (SERMs)** have been developed that are antiestrogenic and have antiresorptive effects on bone.
- **Calcitonin** has been used for many years in the prevention and treatment of osteoporosis.
- Other therapies: Anabolic therapies are under study; none is approved for osteoporosis. Intermittent injections of parathyroid hormone and fluoride stimulate bone formation and inhibit bone resorption, but their safety and efficacy remain to be established. Thiazides can decrease urinary calcium excretion and slow bone loss. They may be particularly useful in patients with hypercalciuria and osteoporosis (eg, those with idiopathic hypercalciuria).

8. *PHYSIOLOGY OF PREGNANCY*

Definition of pregnancy:- the period from conception to birth of the baby. After the egg is fertilized by a sperm and then implanted in the lining of the uterus, it develops in to the placenta and embryo and later in the fetus.

Maternal physiology:- the physiological changes that occur in the mother during the pregnancy are as following:-

Vagina:-Vaginal wall becomes more hypertrophied and edematous and vascular. The increased blood supply gives bluish coloration of the mucosa .The secretions become more thin, curdy white and copious.

Vulva:- Vulva becomeedematous and hyperemic, superficial varicosities may appear.

Uterus:- In the non pregnant state the weight of uterus is about 50 grams but in pregnancy it is 900-1000 grams, and length increase from 7.5 cm to 35 cm. The muscles become hypertrophied occurs due to the influence of the estrogen and progesterone releasing during the pregnancy.

Inthe pregnant state the uterus is supplied by the uterine, ovarian supply and via lymphatic supply most pronounced at the placental site.

Shapeof uterus: In non pregnant it is in pyriform , globular at 12 weeks ,oval by 28 and spherical at 38 weeks of gestation.

Position of uterus:- Normally uterus is in anteverted position up to 8 weeks afterwards it becomes erect in the position.

Cervix:- There is the hypertrophy and hyperplasia of the elastic and connective tissues, vascularity increased which leads to the softening of the cervix (Goodell's sign) evident at 6 weeks cervical secretions become thick and copious known as leucorrhea of pregnancy.

Ovaries:- There is the persistent growth of the corpus luteum which reaches the maximum at 8 week and it measures about 2.5 cm. It looks bright orange later becomes yellow and finally appears in pallor. Hormones estrogen and progesteron maintain the environment for the growing ovum before the action taken over by the placenta.

Breasts: - The changes in the breast are more evident in the primi mothers. The size increase due to the marked hypertrophy and proliferation of the ducts and the alveoli. Vascularity is increased which result in appearance of bluish veins running under the skin. Nipples become larger and erectile and deeply pigmented. The sebaceous glands and the areola become hypertrophied. An irregular pigmented areola appears during the 2nd trimester called secondary areola.

The secretions can be squeezed out of the breast at about 12 weeks of the pregnancy which at 1st becomes sticky by 16 weeks become thick and yellowish.

Cutaneous changes:- The distribution of pigmentory changes is selective.

- **Face:**) it is an extreme form of pigmentation around the cheeks, forehead, and around the eyes. It may be patchy or diffuse, disappears soon after the delivery.
- **Breast:** Bluish coloration around the nipple known as the secondary areola.
- **Linea Nigra:-** It is the brownish black pigmented area in the midline stretching from the xiphisternum to the symphysis pubis due to the effect of the hormones disappears soon after the delivery.
- **Striae Gravidarum:-** They are predominantly found in the abdominal wall and below the umbilicus. They are pinkish in beginning but after delivery it becomes glistening white in appearance and is known as striae albicans.

Weight Gain:- The total weight gain in a healthy pregnancy is averages 11 kg. It is distributed as following:-

Reproductive weight gain as follows:

- Fetus :- 3.3 kg
- Placenta :- 600 grams
- Liquor :-800 grams
- Uterus :- 900 grams
- Breasts :-400 grams

Net maternal weight gain:-

- Accumulation of the fat and protein:- 3.5 kg
- Increase in the extra cellular blood fluid:- 1.2 kg
- Increased blood volume:- 1.3 kg

Body water metabolism:- During the pregnancy, the amount of water at term remains about 6.5 liters. Water content of fetus, placenta and amniotic fluid is about 3.5 liters . Pregnancy is a state of the hypervolemia . There is the active retention of the sodium, potassium and water.

Haematological changes:-

Blood volume:- During the pregnancy there is the increased vascularity of the enlarging uterus with the interposition of utero-placental circulation

Heart and circulation:- A systolic murmur may be audible in the apical or pulmonary area.

Cardiac output it is lowest in the sitting and supine position and highest in the right or left or knee chest position. It reaches at the peak 40-50% at about by 30-32 weeks.

It is caused by the following factors.

- Increased blood volume
- To meet the required oxygen due to the increased metabolic activity.

Blood Pressure: - The systolic blood pressure will be 110-120 mm/hg and diastolic remains at 65-80 mm/hg.

Respiratory system:- With the enlargement of the uterus specially in the later month there is the elevation of the diaphragm and breathing become diaphragmatic and respiratory rate is 40breaths/minute. **Musculoskeletal changes**:- Varicose vein, Cramps of the muscles, may develop. Spine curve increases leads to the back pain and pain in the shoulder area.

Nervous System: - Nausea, vomiting, mental irritability and sleepiness due to the psychological factors.

Urinary system: - **Bladder** irritability and frequency of micturition are more common.

Digestive system:- Gum may become spongy and bleed to touch. , due to the regurgitation of the HCl from the stomach. Heart burn may occur and atomicity of the gut leads to the constipation .Liver function may be depressed.

Metabolic system:- Total metabolic changes occur due to growing fetus and uterus. Basal metabolic rate is increase to the extent of 30% higher than the non pregnant state.

- **Protein metabolism:** - There is the positive nitrogenous balance throughout the pregnancy. At term the fetus and placenta contains about 500 gm of protein.
- **Carbohydrate metabolism:-** Insulin secretion is increased in response to glucose and amino acids. There is the hyperplasia and hypertrophy of the beta cells of the pancreas. Sensitivity of the insulin increased due to the number of contra insulin factors.(estrogen, progesterone , human placental lactogen)
- **Fat metabolism:** - An average of 3-4 4 kg of fat is stored during the pregnancy mostly in the abdominal wall, hips and thighs and breasts .Plasma lipids and lipoproteins increases during the later half of pregnancy.
- **Lipid metabolism:** - HDL level increase by 15%. The activity of the lipoprotein lipase is increased.
- **Iron metabolism:-**Iron is absorbed in the ferrous form, the placenta to the fetus. Total iron requirement is estimated as 1000 mg.

Diagnostic Evaluation of the pregnancy:-

The reproductive period of the woman begins at the menarcheand ends with the menopause that extends from 13-45 years.

Diagnosis for the 1st trimester

- **Subjective symptoms :-**

    ○ **Amenorrhea** during the reproductive period previously having the normal period is considered to be the pregnancy. However cyclic pregnancy may occur up to the 12th week, until the decidual space is obliterated by the fusion of the decidua vera with decidua capsularis.

This type of bleeding is usually scanty, lasting for a shorter duration of time must not be confused with the pathological problem like abortion.
- **Morning sickness** is consistently present in the 50% cases., more often in the 1st pregnancy. It usually appears soon after the missed period and last beyond the 3rd month. It varies from the nausea to the loss of appetite or even vomiting
- **Frequency of micturition** is due to the rest of the bulky uterus on th e fundus of the bladder, congestion of bladder mucosa, change in osmoregulation cause increased thirst and polyuria.
- **Breast discomfort** in the form of feeling of fullness and 'pricking sensation' especially in the primigravida mother.
- **Fatigue** is the frequent symptom which may occur early in the pregnancy.

- Objective symptoms:-

    - The breast changes are more evident in the primi mothers. Montogomery tubercles are more evident. Thick yellowish secretions can be expressed by 12 weeks.
    - **Per Abdomen:-** Uterus remains a pelvic organ until 12 weeks
    - **Pelvic changes:-**
    - **Jacquemier's or Chadwick sign:-** It is the discoloration of the vaginal wall due to the local vascular congestion visible at about 8th week.
    - **Vaginal sign:-** In this the anterior vaginal wall becomes soft, copious mucous discharge and the pulsation felt at the lateral fornics at 8th week called Osiander's sign.
    - **Cervical sign:-** Cervix becomes soft as early as 6th week, the pregnant cervix feels like the lip of the mouth and non pregnant cervix is like the tip of the nose.

On speculum examination the bluish discoloration is visible due to te increased vascularity.

- **Uterine sign:-** The uterus is enlarges to the shape of hen egg at 6th week, size of cricket ball at 8th week and size of fetal head at 12 weeks. The pregnant uterus feels soft and elatic.

- **IMMUNOLOGICAL TEST FOR PREGNANCY:-**

Schematic representation of immunological tests
Pregnant
Urine + HCG
(containing hcg) Antiserum

- Neutrilisation of the antibody
- Hcg coated latex particles
- No visible agglutination

Non- Pregnant
Urine + HCG
(no hcg) Antiserum

- Hcg antibodies not neutralised
- Hcg coated latex particles
- visible agglutination

2) **Enzyme linked immunosorbent assay :-** It is based on the monoclonal antibody
That binds the hcg and the second antibody that is linked with the enzyme alkaline phosphate .It is detected by colour changes, can detect the hcg within 5 days of missed period.

Ultrasonography:- Intradecidual sac is identified in between 25-30 days of gestation.

Second trimester:-
Symptoms:- Nausea, vomiting, frequency of micturition usually subsides but amenorrhea continuous.

- **Quickening :-** it denotes the perception of active fetal movements by the woman, usually felt by the 8th week
- Progressive enlargement of the lower abdomen due to the growing fetus.
- General examination includes choasma and breast changes.
- Abdominal examination :- linea nigra and striae observed on the inspection.

  - **Palpation includes the following changes:-**

- Uterus feels soft and elastic and oval in shape
- Braxton-Hick contraction are evident
- Palpation of fetal parts by 20th week
- Active fetal movements can be felt byy palacing the hand over the uterus

  - **Auscultation:-** Fetal heart sound is the most conclusive sign of the pregnancy. With the help of the stethoscope it can be detected by 18-20 weeks. The rate varies from 140-160 beats per minute.
  - **Last trimester:-** Symptoms :- Amenorrhea persists.

Enlargement of abdomen continuous.

- Lightening at about 38 weeks
- Frequancy of micturition reappears
- Fetal movements are more pronounced.

Signs:-

- Cutaneous changes more prominent.
- Uterine shape change to spherical.
- Fundal height increased.
- Braxton – Hick contractions are more evident.
- Fetal movements are easily felt.
- Ultrasonography in last trimester.

FOETAL PHYSIOLOGY AND COMPLICATION

FETUS; in humans, the unborn young from the end of 8th week after conception to movement of birth, as different from earlier embryo is called as fetus. PHYSIOLOGY of NUTRITION; there are three stages of fetal nutrition are;

1. ABSORPTION; in the early post fertilization period nutrition is stored in the dutoplasm within the cytoplasm and very little extra nutrition is supplied from uterine secretions.

2. HISTOTROPHIC TRANSFER; before the establishment of utero-placental circulation the nutrition is derived from decidua by diffusion.

3. HAEMATOTROPHIC; with establishment of fetal circulation nutrition is obtained by active and passive transfer from third week onward.

FOETAL CIRCULATION; There are three shunts in fetal circulation are:

1.Ductus arteosis; it protect the lungs against circulation overload and allow the right ventricle to strength the pulmonary vascular resistance, it carries mostly oxygen saturated Blood.

2. DUCTOUS VENOSUS; Fetal vessels connecting umbilical vein to caudal vena cava and blood flow is regulated by spincher, it carries mostly high oxygenated blood.

3. FORANEN OVALE; it is an opening between the two atria enabling blood to channelize directly into systematic circulation thereby bypassing the lungs.

- UMBLICAL ARTERY; it is a paired artery that is found in the pelvic and abdominal region and extend into umbilical cord.
- UMBLICAL VEIN; is a large red vessel at the far left. Umbilical arteries wrap around the umbilical vein
- FETAL BLOOD; site of blood formation are first in yolk sac then fetal liver and lastly in bone marrow. Anti-A and Anti- B appear in the fetal blood at about 4-8 months after the birth. Blood cells are; ERYTHROCYTES- All are nucleated at term only number is 6 million/ mm3
- HAEMOGLOBIN; 15-20 mg/dl at term
- SERUM IRON; 150gm/dl at term
- LEUKOCYTIC COUNT; at term 2-3 times the adult one
- RHESHUS FACTOR; can be detected in fetal blood from 10 week
- SKIN; at the 16 week languo appear but near term almost completely disappear. Sebaceous glands appear at 20th week and sweat gland somewhat later. horny layer of epidermis is absent before 20 week.
- **RESPIRATORY SYSTEM;** respiration can be detected at the 11th week with help of ultrasound. From the beginning of 4th month respiratory movement is sufficient to move the amniotic fluid in and out the respiratory tract.
- **DIGESTIVE SYSTEM;**

INTESTINE; the small intestine undergoes peristalsis by 11th week of gestation.

FETAL SWALLOWING; from 2nd trimester fetal swallow and absorb the amniotic fluid.

MECONIUM; it consist of undigested debris from the swallowed amniotic fluid secretions and desquamation from gastrointestinal tract.

LIVER; conjugation of free billirubin is limited, glycogen appear in low concentration but near the term it appear 2-3 times those in adult liver.

GALL BLADDER; it secrete bile from 3rt month of gestation.

PANCREASE; it respond to hyperglycemia by increasing insulin secretions.

URINART SYSTEM; by the end of 1st trimester the kidneys can excrete urine which is hypotonic due to low electrolytes concentration. Full fetal bladder can be seen by ultrasound.

CENTRAL NERVOUS SYSTEM; at full term partially developed and functioned. By the end of the 1st yr of life the brain doubles its weight.

ENDOCRINE GLAND;1. ANTERIOR PITUTARY; before the end of 17th week, the fetal pituitary is able to synthesis and store all pituitary hormones (thyroid and parathyroid glands).they are capable to function by the end of first trimester

ADRENAL GLAND; outer zone of fetal adrenal cortex produce cortisol and inner zone produce dehydropaindrosterone, adrenal medulla produce small amount of catecholamine.

GONADS; testosterone is synthesized by the fetal testis from progesterone. Estrogen is synthesized by fetal ovaries.

FOETAL COMPLICATIONS;

- CONGENITAL MALFORMATION; risk of congenital malformation increase in the mothers suffer to diabetes mellitus.
- BIRTH WEIGHT AND ADIPOSITY; fetal hyperinsulemia occur due to maternal hyperglycemia. Maternal overweight and obesity is an additional risk for this.
- MALPRESENTATION; condition in which the fetus and baby is not in head down position in uterus and baby is positioned down buttocks and head-ups.
- ECTOPIC PREGNANCY; implantation of embryo outside the uterus, it occur due to smoking, advance ,maternal age and prior damage of fallopian tubes.
- PLACENTAL ABRUPTION; Separation of placenta from uterus, risk factors are maternal hypertension, trauma and drug use.

- SPONTANEOUS ABORTION; abortion may be occur due to infection.

9. URINARY INCONTINENCE

Urinary incontinence is defined as the involuntary loss of urine from the bladder.

Incidence

More than 17 million adults in United States are estimated to have urinary incontinence.

It affects people of all ages but is particularly common among the elderly.

Risk factors for urinary incontinence

- Pregnancy: Vaginal delivery, episiotomy.
- Menopause
- Genitourinary surgery
- Pelvic muscle weakness
- Incompetent urethra due to trauma or sphincter relaxation.
- Immobility
- High impact exercises
- Diabetes mellitus
- Stroke
- Age related changes in the urinary tract
- Morbid obesity
- Cognitive disturbances: Dementia, Parkinson's disease.
- Medications: Diuretics, sedatives, hypnotics, opioids.
- Caregiver or toilet unavailable.

Types of incontinence

- **Stress incontinence**

It is the involuntary loss of urine through an intact urethra as a result of sneezing, coughing, or changing position.

It predominantly affects women who have had vaginal deliveries and thought to be the result of decreasing ligament and pelvic floor support of the urethra and decreasing or absent estrogen levels within the urethral walls and bladder base.

In men, often after a radical prostatectomy for prostate cancer because of loss of urethral compression that the prostate had supplied before the surgery, and possibly bladder wall irritability.

- **Urge incontinence**

It is the involuntary loss of urine associated with a strong urge to void that cannot be suppressed. The patient is aware of the need to void but is unable to reach the toilet in time.

An uninhibited detrusor contraction is the precipitating factor.

This can occur in patient with neurologic dysfunction that impairs inhibition of bladder contraction.

- **Reflex incontinence**

It is involuntary loss of urine due to hyperreflexia in the absence of normal sensation usually associated with voiding.

This commonly occurs in patient with spinal cord injury because they have neither neurologically mediated motor control of the detrusor nor sensory awareness of the need to void.

- **Overflow incontinence**

It is involuntary loss of urine associated with over distension of the bladder.

Such over distension result from the bladder inability to empty normally despite frequent urine loss. Neurologic abnormalities and factor that obstruct outflow of urine can cause overflow incontinence.

- **Functional incontinence**

It refer to those conditions in which lower urinary tract function is intact but other factor such as severe cognitive impairment, make it difficult for the patient to identify the need to void or physical impairment make it difficult to reach to the toilet in time.

- **Iatrogenic incontinence**

It refers to the involuntary loss of urine due to extrinsic medical factors.eg. Use of alpha adrenergic agent o decrease blood pressure. These agents adversely affect the alpha receptors responsible for bladder neck closing pressure, the bladder neck relax to the point of incontinence with a minimal increase in intra abdominal pressure then cause incontinence. When medication is discontinued the incontinence resolve.

Assesment and diagnostic findings

- History collection:- it includes detailed description of the problem and history of medication used.
- The patient voiding history, a diary of fluid intake and output.
- Urodynamic test
- Urinanalysis and urine culture

Medical management

- Behavioural therapy
- Pharmacologic therapy
- Surgical management

Behavioral therapy: - These therapies are the 1st choice to decrease or eliminate urinary incontinence. it include :-

- pelvic floor muscle exercise (kegal exercises)
- voiding diary
- bio feedback
- verbal instructions
- physical therapy

Pharmacologic therapy:-

- Anticholinergic agent inhibits bladder contraction and is considered first line medication for urge incontinence.
- Tricyclic antidepressant medication e.g amoxapine can also decrease bladder contraction as well as increase bladder neck resistance.
- Stress incontinence may be treated with pseudoephedrine sulphate, which acts on alpha-adrenergic receptors.

- Hormone therapy (e g .estrogen) taken orally, transdermally, topically was once the treatment of choice for urinary incontinence in postmenopausal women. Estrogen is believed to decrease obstruction to urine flow by restoring the mucosal integrity of the urethra.

Surgical Management

Surgical correction indicated to patients who have not achieved continence using behavioral and pharmacological therapy.

- Lifting or stabilizing the bladder or urethra to restore the normal urethrovesical angel or lengthen the urethra.
- Women with stress incontinence may undergo an anterior vaginal repair or needle suspension to reposition the urethra.
- Procedure to compress the urethra and increase the resistance to urine flow include sling procedures and placement of periurethral bulking agents such as artificial collagens.
- Periurethral bulking is a semi permanent procedure in which small amounts of artificial collagen fibers are placed within the walls of the urethra to enhance the closing pressure of the urethra.
- An artificial urinary sphincter can also be used to close the urethra and promote continence. Two types of artificial sphincters are

i. A periurethral cuff and
ii. A cuff inflation pump.

10. *UTERINE PROLAPSE*

Uterine prolapse is abnormal position of the uterus in which the uterus protrudes downward.

Risk factors: - long second stage of labour
-increased abdominal pressure
- Genetic predisposition to weakness in connective tissue
-obesity
- Prior pelvic surgery

Degree of prolapse:

- **First degree** – the cervix drops into the vagina

- **Second degree-** The cervix drops to the level just inside the opening of the vagina
- **Third degree-** The cervix is outside the vagina
- **Fourth degree-** The entire uterus is outside the vagina.

Causes: Failure to support pelvic organ
Congenital: due to weakness of pelvic support
Acquired:

a] stretching and tearing of pelvic muscles or ligaments during child birth.

b] Early bearing down (before dilation of cervix)

c) Early delivery of head without emptying bladder.

d) Atrophy of pelvic floor support in menopause with under nutrition.

e) Chronic pelvic inflammatory disease that effect to ligaments

f) Multipara women

g) Pressure of chronic cough, constipation, heavy weight lifting and obesity.

Associated conditions:

1. **Cystocele :** cystocele is a downward displacement of the bladder towards the vaginal orifice resulting from damage to the anterior vaginal support structures
2. **Enterocele –** The herniation of the upper rear vaginal wall where a small bowel portion bulges into the vagina.
3. **Rectocele:** The herniation of the lower rear vaginal wall where the rectum bulges into the vagina.

Sign and symptoms:
- Patient complain of something coming per vagina
- sacral and lumber pain
- Backache
- White discharge per vagina
- Ulceration of cervix
- Poor health
- Anaemia

Effects: A) On pregnancy :
1) There is an increased chance of abortion.

4. Discomfort due to increased ailments
5. Premature rupture of the membranes
6. Intrauterine infection

B) During labour;
1) Early rupture of the membrane
2) Cervical dystocia
3) Prolonged labour due to non-dilation of cervix

Diagnostic Evaluation: 1) History collection

- Patient should be examined carefully on basis of physical examination
- Make the patient to cough and strain and note the nature and degree of prolapsed.
- Perineal musceles are palpate and examine for muscle tone
- Check Hb.

Management;
Medical Management:

- **1) Kegel exercise** – Which involve contracting or tightening the vaginal muscles are prescribed to help strengthen these weakened muscles.
- **2) Pessaries** can be used to avoid surgery. This device is inserted into the vagina and positioned to keep an organ, such as the bladder, uterus, or intestine, properly aligned when a cystocele , rectocele , or prolapsed has occurred.Pesseries are usually ring shaped and are made various material such as rubber or plastic . The size and type of pessary are selected and fitted by a gynecologic health care provider.

11. *EXERCISE PRESCRIPTION FOR HEART DISEASE*

- Cardiovascular diseases are steadily emerging as the number one killer worldwide; the implications are even more significant in India.
- There were predicated 3.75 million deaths due to cardiovascular disease in 2010 across the country. Out of which 2 million deaths were due to heart attacks or coronary artery disease.

Principles of cardiac rehab

- Enable the patient to regain full physical, psychological and social status.
- Promote secondary prevention to optimise long term prognosis.
- Comprehensive cardiac rehabilitation.

Contra-indications

- Unstable angina.
- Resting BP> 200/110mmhg.
- Orthostastic BP drop >20mmhg.
- Uncompensated CHF.
- Uncontrolled diabetes.
- Active pericarditis.
- Resting ST segment displacement>2mm.

Cardiac Rehabilitation Goals
The goal is to improve or maintain a good level of cardiovascular fitness.
- For those able to return to work:
1. Return to productive employment as soon as possible
2. Improve and maintain as good cardiovascular fitness
- For those not able to return to work:
1. Maintain as active a life as possible
2. Establish new areas of interest to improve quality of life
- Patient Education and Reduction of Coronary Risk Factors.

Core components of Cardiac Rehab

- Patient assessment
- Nutritional counseling
- Lipid management
- Hypertension management
- Smoking cessation
- Diabetes management
- Psychosocial management
- General education (meds, procedures, condition)
- Physical activity counseling
- Exercise training

Rationale for Cardiac rehab
1. Early ambulation

2. Exercise training
3. Secondary prevention
4. Education

Phases

Phase I (acute phase or monitoring phase) - In-patient stay

Phase II (subacute or rehabilitation phase) - Post discharge at home, (2 – 6 weeks)

Phase III (training or intensive rehab) - Out-patient care, Delivered by health care services. (6 -12 weeks)

Phase IV (ongoing conditioning or phase) - Long term, Delivered by leisure services.

- **Exercise Intensity**

Exercise intensity is usually prescribed as some percentage of the maximum capacity obtained on exercise testing, (i.e., O2 consumption, heart rate workload and/or degree of exertion)

- *O2 Consumption*
- Threshold 40–50% max VO2 60% max HR
- Optimum 55–65% max VO2 70% max HR
- For the deconditioned cardiac patient, exercise even at 40% to 50% of max VO2 will result in improvement
- **Target Heart Rate (THR)**
- Exercise intensity is based on target heart rate
- Note: Clearance Heart Rate (HR) is the clinical maximum HR attained on stress test.
- Target HR is the following range:
- Clearance HR × .7 = beginning range
- Clearance HR × .85 = end range
- 1. For the cardiac patient, 70% of the maximum HR attained on the exercise stress test
- 2. For the healthy patient, 70% to 85% of the predicted age-adjusted maximum HR
- **Duration and Frequency of Exercise**
- The duration depends on the level of fitness of the individual and the intensity of the exercise

- The usual duration when exercise is at 70% of maximum heart rate is 20–30 minutes at conditioning level
- In the poorly conditioned individual, daily exercise as low as 3–5 minutes can bring about improvement. For the conditioned individual who prefers to exercise at higher intensities, duration of exercise may be reduced to 10–15 minutes

Exercise considerations for the angina patient

- Goal: increase anginal and ischemic threshold.
- Prolonged warm-up & cool down (gradual rise).
- Target HR below ischmic level (± 10 bpm)
- Caution with exertion in the cold.
- Upper body exercise may precipitate symptoms due to higher pressure response.
- Monitor blood pressures before and after exercise.
- Alternative exercise: frequent, short, intermittent sessions.

Exercise considerations for the CHF patient

- Must be on stable medical therapy
- Monitor hypokalemia and hemodynamic response
- Malignant dysrhythmia
- THR 40-70% VO2max 3-7days per week, 20-40 minutes per session
- Long warm-up and cool down
- Interval exercise training.

Exercise considerations for the pacemaker

- Monitor systolic pressures
- Extended warm-up and cool down
- Rate modulated pacemakers intensity:
  - Karvonen method
  - RPE
  - METs

Exercise considerations for the CABG

- ROM and mobility exercises
- Light hand weights
- Stretching and flexibility
- Avoid resistance training until sternum healed (3 months)
- Initial aerobic training (resting HR +30bpm)
- Valve patients: longer recovery, slower rate, more limitations

Cardiovascular Risk Factors Based On Priority for Intervention

Class 1: Factors for which interventions have proved to lower coronary artery disease risk.
 - Cigarette smoking
 - High LDL cholesterol
 - High fat/cholesterol diet
 - Hypertension
 - Left Ventricular Hypertrophy
 - Thrombogenic factors

Class 2: Factors for which interventions are likely to lower coronary artery disease risk.
 - Diabetes Mellitus
 - Physical inactivity
 - Low LDL cholesterol
 - High triglycerides; small dense LDL
 - Obesity
 - Postmenopausal status (women)

Class 3: Factors that if modified might lower coronary artery disease risk

- Psychosocial factors

  - Lipoprotein (a)
  - Homocysteine
  - Oxidative stress

- No alcohol consumption

Class 4: Factors that cannot be modified or for which modification would be used would be unlikely to lower coronary artery disease risk.
 - Age

- Male Gender
- Low socioeconomic status
- Family history of early onset CVD

12. EXERCISE AND DIABETES

- Diabetes mellitus is a clinical syndrome characterized by hyperglycemias caused by absolute or relative deficiency of insulin.
- Type 1: T cell mediated autoimmune disease involving destruction of insulin-secreting beta cells in pancreatic islets which takes place over many years. Classical symptoms of diabetes occur only when 70-90% of beta cells have been destroyed.
- Type 2: more complex than diabetes 1 because there is a combination of resistance to actions of insulin in liver and muscle together with impaired pancreatic beta cell function leading to relative insulin deficiency.
- Insulin resistance.
- Pancreatic beta cell failure.

Exercise in Type 1 Diabetes

- Control of blood glucose is achieved in a patient with type 1 DM through a balance in the carbohydrate intake, exercise level and insulin dosage.
- Meal and exercise should be adjusted according to the patients' response.
- Frequent self monitoring should occur, until a balance is achieved among diet, exercise and insulin parameters.
- The ideal pre-exercise blood level is 6.6-10 mmol/L.
- The athletes who have blood glucose concentrations exceeding 11 mmol/L and ketones and the urine, should postpone exercise and take supplemental insulin.
- Those with blood glucose level less than 5.5 mmol/L requires pre-exercise carbohydrate snack.
- Exercise for 20-30 min at less than 70% VO2max requires a rapidly absorbable carbohydrate before exercise but needs minimal insulin dosing adjustments.
- More vigorous activity of less than 1 hour often requires a 25% reduction in pre-exercise insulin and 15-30g of rapidly absorbed carbohydrate exchange before and every 30 min after the onset of activity

- Strenuous activity of longer than 1 hour will require a 30-80% reduction in pre-exercise insulin and ingestion of two fruit exchange every 30 min.
- After exercise hyperglycemia will occur, but insulin should still be decreased by 25-50% (because insulin sensitivity is increased for 12-15 hours after activity has ceased).
- Consuming carbohydrate within 30 min after exhaustive, glycogen-depleting exercise allows for more efficient restoration of muscle glycogen.
- This will help to prevent post-exercise, late-onset hypoglycemia.

Exercise in Type 2 Diabetes

- Those patients with type 2 diabetes who are managed with diet therapy alone do not usually need to make any adjustments for exercise.
- Patients taking oral hypoglycemic drugs may need to halve their dose on days of prolonged exercise or withhold them altogether, depending on their blood glucose levels. Advised to carry glucose with them.

Benefits of exercise
Benefits of type 1 diabetics:

- Improved insulin sensitivity
- Improved blood lipid profile
- Decreased heart rate and blood pressure at rest
- Decreased body weight
- Decreased risk of coronary heart disease
- Insulin requirement may decrease slightly.

In type 2 diabetes

- A program of regular physical activity can reverse many of the defects in metabolism of both fat and glucose that occur in people with type 2 diabetes.
- HbA1C is used as an index of long term blood glucose control. The lower the value, the better. HbA1C reduced by chronic exercise in people with type 2 DM.

Diabetes and competition

- Diabetic athletes participate in team sport should know about the normal glucose profile.
- Good control of blood glucose levels may requires regular access to carbohydrate containing drinks
- This not only serves to improve glucose profile but also aids rehydration during prolonged exercise.

Diabetes and travel

- They should carry insulin, needles and blood glucose testing equipment.
- Copies of prescriptions should be taken.
- Travel from north to south generally requires no alteration to insulin doses.
- East to west travel of more than 5 hours requires insulin dose adjustment.
- They should check blood glucose levels at least every 6 hours on the flight.

High-risk sports

- Hypoglycemic attacks, characterized by lack of concentration.
- Sports such as: mountain climbing, sky diving, scuba diving should be avoided.

Exercise and the complications of diabetes

- Poor glucose control appears to be associated with increase occurrence of neuropathy.
- Abnormal autonomic function is common among those with diabetes of long duration.
- The risk of exercise when autonomic neuropathy is present include: hypoglycemia, abnormal heart rate, blood pressure response, impaired sympathetic and parasympathetic activity and abnormal thermoregulation.
- High intensity activity should be avoided. Water activity and stationary cycling are recommended.
- For peripheral neuropathy: correct footwear, regular close inspection of feet, feet and toes should be kept dry and clean and non weight bearing

exercises are recommended.
- Exercises that improve balance are of good choice.

Complications of exercise in the diabetic athlete
Hypoglycemia

It is major concern for type 1 DM. The use of too much exogenous insulin will prevent hepatic glucose production, and cause increase glucose uptake into skeletal muscles with subsequent risk of hypoglycemia.

- Initial symptoms: sweating, headache, nervousness, tremor and hunger.
- If not corrected: confusion, abnormal behavior, loss of consciousness and convulsions may occur.
- After indication, the athlete should ingest oral carbohydrate.
- Semiconscious and unconscious requires IV glucose administration.
- Athletes usually requires to 15-30g of glucose per half hour of vigorous exercise.

Diabetic ketoacidosis in the athlete

- Despite increased glucose uptake that occurs in exercise independent of insulin, a relative deficiency of insulin can lead to hyperglycemia, hyperlipidemia and possible ketoacidosis.
- Individual with blood glucose level of 20-30mmol/L and above are at high risk of ketoacidosis if exercise vigorously.
- This is because the counter-regulatory hormone response to exercise pushes the glucose levels higher and there is insufficient insulin to prevent ketosis.

Musculoskeletal manifestations of diabetes

- Frozen shoulder.
- Limited joint mobility.
- Carpal tunnel syndrome.
- Flexor tenosynovitis.
- Complex regional pain syndrome type 1.
- Neuropathic joints.

CHAPTER FIVE

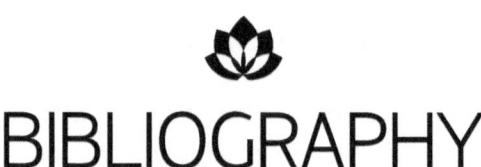

BIBLIOGRAPHY

1. Hayden J, Van Tulder MW, Malmivaara A, Koes BW. Exercise therapy for treatment of non-specific low back pain. Cochrane database of systematic reviews. 2005(3).
2. Assendelft WJ, Morton SC, Emily IY, Suttorp MJ, Shekelle PG. Spinal manipulative therapy for low back pain: a meta-analysis of effectiveness relative to other therapies. Annals of internal medicine. 2003 Jun 3;138(11):871.
3. Cheng RS, Pomeranz B. Electrotherapy of chronic musculoskeletal pain: comparison of electroacupuncture and acupuncture-like transcutaneous electrical nerve stimulation. The Clinical journal of pain. 1986 Jan 1;2(3):143-50.
4. Qing LI. Application of vascular interventional actinotheraphy in gynecologic diseases [J]. Journal of Jinggangshan Medical College. 2003;1.
5. Thiel H. Low power laser therapy—an introduction and a review of some biological effects. The Journal of the Canadian Chiropractic Association. 1986 Sep;30(3):133.
6. Deyle GD, Henderson NE, Matekel RL, Ryder MG, Garber MB, Allison SC. Effectiveness of manual physical therapy and exercise in osteoarthritis of the knee: a randomized, controlled trial. Annals of internal medicine. 2000 Feb 1;132(3):173-81.
7. Threlkeld AJ. The effects of manual therapy on connective tissue. Physical therapy. 1992 Dec 1;72(12):893-902.
8. Geytenbeek J. Evidence for effective hydrotherapy. Physiotherapy. 2002 Sep 1;88(9):514-29.
9. Vaile J, Halson S, Gill N, Dawson B. Effect of hydrotherapy on recovery from fatigue. International journal of sports medicine. 2008

Jul;29(07):539-44.
10. Pountney T. Physiotherapy for children. Elsevier Health Sciences; 2007 Sep 13.
11. Stokes M, Stack E, editors. Physical Management for Neurological Conditions E-Book:[Formerly Physical Management in Neurological Rehabilitation E-Book]. Elsevier Health Sciences; 2011 Apr 19.
12. Stanhope J, Grimmer-Somers K, Milanese S, Kumar S, Morris J. Extended scope physiotherapy roles for orthopedic outpatients: an update systematic review of the literature. Journal of multidisciplinary healthcare. 2012;5:37.
13. de Brito Vieira WH, Aguiar KA, Da Silva KM, Canela PM, Da Silva FS, Abreu BJ. Overview of ultrasound usage trends in orthopedic and sports physiotherapy. Critical ultrasound journal. 2012 Dec;4(1):11.
14. Matte P, Jacquet L, Van Dyck M, Goenen M. Effects of conventional physiotherapy, continuous positive airway pressure and non-invasive ventilatory support with bilevel positive airway pressure after coronary artery bypass grafting. Acta Anaesthesiologica Scandinavica. 2000 Jan;44(1):75-81.
15. Dalal HM, Doherty P, Taylor RS. Cardiac rehabilitation. Bmj. 2015 Sep 29;351:h5000.
16. Hesse KA, Campion EW. Motivating the geriatric patient for rehabilitation. Journal of the American Geriatrics Society. 1983 Oct;31(10):586-9.
17. Brukner P. Brukner & Khan's clinical sports medicine. North Ryde: McGraw-Hill; 2012.
18. O'Sullivan SB, Schmitz TJ, Fulk G. Physical rehabilitation. FA Davis; 2019 Jan 25.
19. Houglum PA. Therapeutic Exercise for Musculoskeletal Injuries 4th Edition. Human Kinetics; 2016 May 18.
20. Miller, G. T. (1992). Living in the environment: an introduction to environment science. Wadsworth Publishing Company.
21. Kargarfard, M., Rouzbahani, R., Rezanejad, S., & Poursafa, P. (2009). The Effect of Air Pollution on Cardio Respiratory Performance of Active Individuals. ARYA Atheroscler, 5(2).
22. Hajian, M., & Mohaghegh, S. (2014). Indoor Air Pollution in Exercise Centers. International Journal of Medical Toxicology and Forensic Medicine, 5(1 (winter)), 22-31.

23. A J Carlisle et al. Exercise and outdoor ambient air pollution. Br J Sports Med 2001;35:214-222 doi:10.1136/bjsm.35.4.214
24. Pribyl, C. R., & Racca, J. (1996). Toxic gas exposures in ice arenas. Clinical Journal of Sport Medicine, 6(4), 232-236.
25. Linn WS, Venet TG, Shamoo DA, et al. Respiratory effects of sulfar dioxide in heavily exercising asthmatics. Am Rev Respir Dis1983; 127:278–83.
26. Bevan MAJ, Procter CJ, Baker-Rogers J, et al. Exposure to carbon monoxide, respirable suspended particulates and volotile organic compounds. Environ Sci Technol1991; 25:788–91.
27. Brukner P. Brukner & Khan's clinical sports medicine. North Ryde: McGraw-Hill; 2012.
28. Ades PA. Cardiac Rehabilitation and Secondary Prevention of Coronary Heart Disease. New England Journal of Medicine. *2001 Sep 20;345(12):892-902.*
29. Ayala C et al. Receipt of cardiac rehabilitation services among heart attack survivors—19 states and the District of Columbia. Morbid Mortality Weekly. *2003; 52:1072-1075.*
30. Heart *2007; 93: 862-864.*
31. ACSM Guide to *Exercise Rx 7th Edition.*
32. Guidelines for cardiac rehabilitation, 2 ed,1995.
33. Buckwalter JA, Heckman JD, Petrie DP. An AOA critical issue: aging of the North American population: new challenges for orthopaedics. JBJS. 2003 Apr 1;85(4):748-58.
34. O'Connor FG, Sallis R, Wilder R, Pierre PS. Sports Medicine: Justs the Facts. McGraw Hill Professional; 2004 Aug 22.
35. Buckwalter JA, Heckman JD, Petrie DP: Aging of the North American population: New challenges for Orthopaedics. *J Bone Joint Surg* 85:748–758, 2003.
36. Mengelkock LJ, Pollock ML, Limacher MC et al: Effects of age, physical training, and physical fitness on coronary heart disease risk factors in older track athletes at twenty-year followup. *J Am Geriatr Soc* 45:1446–1453, 1997
37. Maharam LG, Bauman PA, Kalman D et al: Master athletes: Factors affecting performance. *Sports Med* 28:273–285, 1999.
38. Pollock ML, Foster C, Knapp D et al: Effect of age and training on aerobic capacity and body composition of master athletes. *J Appl Physiol* 62:725–731, 1987.

39. Pollock ML, Mengelkoch LJ, Graves JE et al: Twenty-year follow-up of aerobic power and body composition of older track athletes. *J Appl Physiol* 82:1508–1516, 1997.
40. Rock CL: Nutrition of the older athlete. *Clin Sport Med* 10:445–457, 1991. Rogers MA, Hagberg JM, Martin WH et al: Decline in VO2max with aging in master athletes and sedentary men. *J Appl Physiol* 68:2195–2199, 1990.
41. Menard D, Stanish WD: The aging athlete. *Am J Sports Med* 17:187–196, 1989.
42. Kallinen M, Alen M: Sports-related injuries in elderly men still active in sports. *Br J Sports Med* 28:52–55, 1994.
43. Kallinen M, Markku A: Aging, physical activity and sports injuries: An overview of common sports injuries in the elderly. *Sport Med* 20:41–52, 1995.
44. Kannus P, Niittymaki S, Jarvinen M et al: Sports injuries in elderly athletes: A three-year prospective, controlled study. *Age Aging* 18:263–270, 1989.
45. Booth FW, Gordon SE, Carlson CJ et al: Waging war on modern chronic diseases: Primary prevention through exercise biology.*J Appl Physiol* 88:774–787, 2000.
46. Fiatarone-Singh MA: Exercise comes of age: Rationale and recommendations for a geriatric exercise prescription. *J Gerontology: Med Sci* 57A:M262–M282, 2002.
47. Seruga, 1996; Doping control in sports medicine; Aug;18(4):471-6.

www.ingramcontent.com/pod-product-compliance
Lightning Source LLC
Chambersburg PA
CBHW030817180526
45163CB00003B/1320